W9-BLD-960

WELLNESS
ON THE GO

Take the Plunge - It's Your Life!

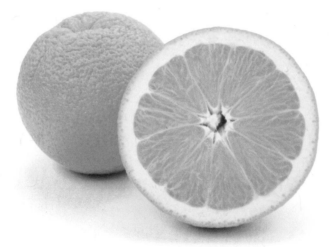

DR. NATHALIE BEAUCHAMP, B.SC., D.C
ANDRÉE J. BENSON, BA ADULT ED. CMIC

Published by:

Baico Publishing Inc.
294 Albert Street, Suite 103
Ottawa, Ontario K1P 6E6
Tel: (613) 829-5141
E-mail: baico@bellnet.ca
www.baico.ca

Printed by Documents Majemta Inc.

ISBN 978-1-897449-88-2

Table of Contents

In Wellness
Dr. Nathalie & Andrée

health and wellness, which lead me to a Bachelor of Health Science and a Doctor of Chiropractic degree."

Nathalie's interest in health and wellness springs from her own experiences. She explains, "Unfortunately, when I was younger, I became anorexic. To this day, I really don't know why – was it peer pressure or control issues? Regardless of the reasons, what I want to share with readers are my challenges and struggles and how my passion for exercise, nutrition and health probably saved my life."

"I will always remember my volleyball coach sitting me on the bench at a provincial tournament because I was far from a healthy weight and too weak to play. Thanks to him, that was my wake-up call. From then on, I made it my mission to be healthy, well and happy in my own skin and to help others do the same! Has it been easy? No, it is still a work in progress, a journey which I hope the readers will want to take with me!"

To find out more about Dr. Nathalie Beauchamp you can visit her website at www.drnathaliebeauchamp.ca

"Dr. Nathalie Beauchamp is one of the most passionate and energetic people I know. I'm happy she has shared her knowledge and excitement for wellness with us."

Debra Cassera, President, Creating Wellness™ Alliance

Andrée Benson, BA Adult Ed, CMIC

"I believe that everyone has an innate inner wisdom to tap into and by tapping into this wisdom, we can live a spectacular life."

– Andrée J. Benson, BA Adult Ed, CMIC

Andrée is a Certified Integrative Coach and founder of Synergie Leadership, an Executive Training and Coaching company. As a Life and Career Coach, she loves to support her clients in reaching their full potential. She is compassionate, intuitive and very positive. She has had the opportunity of coaching people in all walks of life and assisted them in reaching new heights and greater success in their career and personal lives. Dr. Beauchamp was one of Andrée's first clients.

"When I was going through significant transitions in my life: loss of a job, a divorce and a financial crisis, I was invited to attend The Power Within by an acquaintance. I don't think I even knew what I was doing there. That day, I met Debbie Ford and she became my mentor and teacher. Her wisdom and belief in the power of awareness continue to inspire and motivate me."

Twenty years of progressive experience in the training and professional development industry have given Andrée some deep insights into her coaching work. As a Senior Executive, her business acumen and leadership style supported her in successfully coaching and motivating staff while balancing her responsibilities as a single mom.

"I never stop learning," states Andrée, "and every day brings a new experience, a new adventure to learn from and grow. As a single mom, I have learned to be self-sufficient. As a divorced woman, I have learned to forgive, let go and move on. As a career woman, I have learned the delicate balance of work and play. All of these are gifts! Every day when I coach I trust that I offer these gifts to everyone I meet."

Andrée is authoring a series of children's books using fun and creative stories to bring coaching principles and values to kids from ages five to eight. She has also created a set of affirmation cards which are available on her website, www.synergieleadership.com.

Andrée has enjoyed many exciting careers throughout her life:

- Instructor/Facilitator – Franklin Covey, Forum Learning System
- Actor in TV commercials, theatre – both French and English
- Senior Executive
- Author

"_Grab onto every opportunity to learn, experience and grow!_
Reach beyond the possible!"

– Andrée J. Benson

"Andrée Benson is a masterful and creative coach who loves nothing more than to empower her clients to reach new heights to live a spectacular life. She is inspirational and intuitive."

Dave Scharman, EMBA

Acknowledgments

We are very much aware that without our patients and our clients this book would never have been written. It is through our work with them and our shared experiences that we have learned and grown. Because they have shared their lives and stories with us, we can now share awareness, knowledge and wisdom with others.

Our Deepest Thanks Go Out To:

From Dr Nathalie and Andrée

To our editing team for their dedication to this wonderful project and to the many friends and colleagues who helped us review our book and ensure its quality.

To Carrie Irvine and Bronwyn Hammell, our extraordinary creative team, for the intuitive creation of our cover and for our branding. To Paul Gallipeau, our web designer and our terrific "tech" guy!

To Ray Coderre, president of Baico Publishing: thank you for believing in this book and in our message.

From Andrée

To my son Ben: you are the sunshine of my life, thank you for always trusting that I could accomplish anything I set my mind to. I love you!

To my mom, Marielle: thank you for your unwavering belief in me and for all you have given me.

To my friends, Susan, Ghislaine, Nan, Maria, Cindy, Evelynne, Samantha and David: your unconditional love and support gave me the strength and confidence to see the project through. I am honored to have you in my life.

To Kevin Frost, a great athlete: my deepest gratitude for your willingness to share your story for the book. You continue to be an inspiration.

To Dr. Nathalie, my co-author and chiropractor: without your constant and never-ending quest to find the truth and make things better, this book would not be all that it is.

To Debbie Ford, New York Times best selling author and my mentor: you are my inspiration, without your body of work, from the Secret of the Shadow to the Best Year of Your Life, I would not be where I am today. Thank you, thank you, thank you!

From Dr. Nathalie

To my parents Agathe and Philippe for your constant support: thank you for being my biggest fans! To Stephane, Whitley and Tristan thank you for your patience and understanding with the countless hours spent "upstairs" researching and writing this book.

To my wonderful friends, who listened and encouraged me through the trials and tribulations of writing a book: Deborah, Diane, Julie, Becky, Linda and Chris.

To Andrée, my co-author: thank you for your brilliant idea of writing this book. You never know what you can accomplish until you try!

To Craig Smith and the P99 team for my cool website and amazing ideas and support!

To my dedicated clinic team for your support and encouragement – without you this project would never have been possible: Suzanne, Leslie, Lindsay, Marie, Nadine and Tina.

To my patients who cheered me on every day: this book is for you! Thank you for your inquisitive minds and eagerness to learn. I appreciate your commitment to health and wellness.

To my coach Dr. Michael Gandolfi, who makes me accountable and motivates me to always re-invent myself and reach further. To my "mastermind" wellness team: Deborah MacDonald, Pierre Gaudet, Dr. Mike Reid, Dr. Kahlid Mankal and Dr. Craig Hazel: thank you for your support, energy, purpose and passion.

To Dr. Patrick Gentempo and Debra Cassera, Creating Wellness™ Alliance: thank you for your encouragement and remarkable dedication to help chiropractors bring wellness to their communities.

Introduction

– Andrée and Dr. Nathalie

*"Everything should be made as simple as possible,
but not one bit simpler."*

– Albert Einstein

There is a reason you bought this book. Most likely, you want to feel better – emotionally, physically and spiritually. You may not be able to articulate why exactly, you just know that something is off balance. From our experience in coaching and helping people overcome various challenges in their lives, we have come to discover that all of us want the same basic things – to be healthy, to live a long and happy life, and to have the energy to get there. We're here to tell you that it's possible to have all those things and more. You can achieve peace and tranquility; you can develop a healthier body; you can banish draining, negative thoughts from your mind, and you can create a healthier environment for you, your family and your community.

Welcome to **Wellness on the Go**! We have created this book for people just like you. People for whom life has become a marathon with no finish line in sight; it's for people who are racing around, eating on the run, putting off workouts, slaving on weekends at home and at work, sleep-deprived, stressed out, bummed out and burnt out! And most frightening of all, believing this is the way life is supposed to be! We are like hamsters running, running, running on a wheel in a cage. STOP! What does all this incessant rushing and seeking do to us? Slowly but surely, day by day, it's taking away a bit of our health, a bit of our peace of mind and a bit of our life. We're here to share thoughts, suggestions and steps to take for a new way of life; to highlight a path to a spectacular life!

You are most likely opening this book after a long day at work or perhaps you're on your lunch hour thinking, "I wish I had more time to read and relax." So this could be your first opportunity to STOP, get off of your hamster wheel and take a moment for you ... a small step to changing your life.

At its core, wellness is about living with passion, purpose and a plan ... and having the mind, body and spirit to make that happen. We wanted to write this book because we have found a way to do that in our own lives and we want to share those insights with you. We are bombarded with more and more information about health and wellness today, more than most of us can possibly keep up with. What type of exercise should I do? How can yoga help me? Should I drink tap water or bottled water? Is guilt causing me to stress? Should I be eating organic food? We hear so much about striking a balance, the importance of laughter, and how attitude is everything, but where do we start?

Only you know what your tolerance level is for reading about one more study or hearing one more news report about the dangers of this or that. What we wanted to do in writing this book was to create awareness and simplify some of the information that's out there so you can make more informed choices about what to do to increase your own body, mind and soul's wellness. By reading **Wellness on the Go**, and working through the "*Ask Yourself...*" questions and the "*Your Wellness Strategies*" portion of each chapter, you will be better equipped to understand the latest research and what you plan to do about the information. How you choose to proceed will make a difference in your life and in the lives of your family members. We formulated these exercises to help you consider important issues in your life and help create steps toward a healthier lifestyle.

So how do people get to this place anyway? As we said earlier, there is more information available to us, via the Internet, the news and so on than ever before. We are better educated and more information-savvy than ever. Our bodies, minds and souls have not caught up with the speed at which the information is being pumped out. So we find ourselves in the unpleasant position of feeling unwell, unbalanced, and unhappy. The health system also has difficulty coping ... not only with the information that is surfacing, but also with the demands of our aging population.

Most of us are looking for more natural, self-empowering alternatives. We want to take our mental, physical and spiritual health into our own hands. In **Wellness on the Go**, we suggest that by preventing disease, eating well, exercising, spiritual practice and reducing our inadvertent intake of chemicals (i.e. through the food we eat, cleaning products we use, deodorants we wear or water we drink), we will be able to increase our wellness. The risks of not being well in all three dimensions of health and wellness – physical, psychological and biochemical – can be stress, illness, and disease.

The task of turning our wellness around can seem daunting. You might be thinking, "There are so many things wrong with my life. How the heck can I turn it around? I don't even know where to start." So where can you start? Let's start by taking baby steps, one small step at a time. What do you have to lose? The first step to getting well, in any area of your life, starts with AWARENESS. As cliché as it sounds, we really are what we eat and what we think. Focusing on awareness should be at the core of every decision and every choice we make.

This book will give you the tools and strategies to ask yourself the right questions, and put action plans into motion. This will shift your negative patterns and behaviors and start bringing balance, health and wellness to your life. Remember to start by taking small conscious steps, and as you find your footing, you will most likely increase the number of steps you take and the speed at which you take them.

We want you to use this book as a learning guide and a workbook to engage your mind, body and spirit in the true meaning of health and wellness. The information may seem a bit overwhelming and the wellness strategies tedious. Remember, it's all about balance, so do what you can, when you can. Give yourself the time and space to really absorb what you are reading and consciously decide to move forward at a pace that feels comfortable for you. This is not a race to see who can finish the book the fastest. The kind of awareness and growth we're talking about takes time, but if you invest in yourself, you *will* reap the rewards and live a happier, healthier and more fulfilled life.

We just want to say: "Good for you." You are on your way to an amazing life! Welcome to **Wellness on the Go!**

A Small Gift to Get You on Your Way

You will have noticed already that we included a bookmark for you to use. We have done this for two reasons: the first is to make it easy to find the spot in the book where you left off, and the second reason is to provide you with a gentle reminder to take time to do a short meditation every time you pick up this book. This will help you settle in and relax before absorbing the information we have gathered for you.

Here Are Your Meditation Steps

1. Sit comfortably on a chair or couch and make sure you're in a place where you won't be disturbed and can be alone with your thoughts. Remember to tell your family you are on this journey towards a more balanced lifestyle and that you need this time to yourself – they will reap the benefits too.

2. Next, close your eyes and relax. Take a few slow deep breaths and notice if and where you are holding any tension in your body. If you are, consciously let go of all that tension by breathing out; with every exhale, you are letting the tension fall off you and melt away like snow on a warm spring day.

3. Relax a little more, giving yourself the gift of being in the moment, just for you.

4. Continue breathing normally, focusing on your breath. If thoughts of your day or of stressful matters come to mind, just observe them and then let them go, without judgment. Tell yourself that you will deal with those matters later. For now, just be with yourself, focusing on your breathing, relaxing.

5. Continue breathing normally for a few minutes, allowing yourself to feel at peace. Take a few slow, deep breaths and feel the relaxation and peacefulness sweep over your entire being.

6. When you're ready, open your eyes and be thankful for this moment of peace. You are now ready to start reading and fully integrating what you will learn into your life.

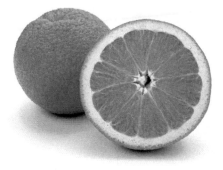

Chapter 1: Listen To Your Body, I Mean *Really* Listen!

– Dr. Nathalie

"Take good care of your body. It's the only place you have to live."
– Jim Rohn

I love to start my weekly health care classes by getting people to think about this question: is it possible for a person to have heart disease, cancer or high blood pressure and not feel any symptoms? In a group setting, where people have come together to learn more about their health and well-being, the answer seems somewhat obvious – yes. As a society, we have been conditioned to mainly respond to symptoms. It's like the old adage, "if it ain't broke, don't fix it!" Many of us think something is wrong with our bodies only when we have symptoms or feel pain!

Take heart attacks, for example. What are the first signs of a heart attack? Most people will answer the standard set of symptoms – chest pain, shortness of breath and numbness in the arm. But what about the heart attacks that are themselves the first symptom without any warning signs? We have all heard about the seemingly healthy guy who goes jogging after work: one minute he's fine and the next he's on the ground! No symptoms. People don't normally develop that kind of heart condition overnight. Was there a genetic predisposition to heart disease that went undetected? What was his overall lifestyle? Did this person have unresolved emotional issues that built up over time causing undue stress and heartache, literally?

What about cancer? Does a person go to bed on a Friday night without cancer and suddenly wake up with it on Saturday morning? Of course not. We may not have felt it, but that does not mean it was not there. Living symptom-free does not necessarily mean we're healthy. Or perhaps, our bodies have gotten so used to feeling a certain way that we no longer feel, or pay attention to what our bodies are desperately trying to tell to us, "Feed me better food! Take me for a walk!" "The stress of this job is really getting to me. The fast food meal I ate again last night has given me a chemical hangover!" It's time to listen!

Signals That Your Body May Be Ailing

While your body won't always give you signals to let you know something is wrong, other times it will be very blunt, so listen up and listen good. Your body is like your car, if the "check engine" light turns on, you could ignore it (for a while) but eventually you go to the garage, right? And if you choose to ignore the signal light, your car may just break down one day, putting you and your passengers at risk.

A good example is a headache, one of the most common ailments in our society today. Health care professionals hear countless patients say that they get "normal" headaches on a frequent basis, but those patients never seem to think there's anything to it, even though there is nothing "normal" about a headache. Even a simple headache is a sign that something is wrong with your body – it could be a neck misalignment, dehydration, low blood sugar, eye strain, poor diet, the list goes on. High blood pressure, heartburn and insomnia are other ailments that many people brush off with a "whatever" attitude; but they too, are serious signs that the body is not working properly.

Health is what happens when your body is functioning optimally. Your nervous system, which is the master system, controls every cell, every tissue and every organ in your body. It has a crucial role in your optimal health. As discussed earlier, pain is not always an indicator that something is wrong. The sensory nerves tell us that there is pain but they only represent approximately 10 percent of our nervous system, which is why symptoms only tell us part of the story. The motor nerves control our muscles, while the autonomic nerves control our internal systems (organs) – both control and coordinate the function of our entire body. Fortunately, many Wellness Chiropractors have technology to measure the function of the nervous system as a whole and do not rely on pain as the only indicator. This state-of-the-art technology provides scans that detect interference in the nervous system. This technology is a great way to measure whether the body is truly working optimally, even if you are not feeling any symptoms.

Unfortunately, many people wait until the car, or in this case their body, breaks down and they reach for the nearest pill to fix the problem. Instead of changing their lifestyle, following a better diet, sticking to an exercise program, or losing the extra 30 pounds that have crept up over the years, they reach for the nearest quick fix. Why? Because popping pills seems a lot easier than taking all of the steps necessary to make a fundamental change in lifestyle. And it's no wonder we're conditioned to reach for pills first; what do we see on television every single day? Got a headache? Pop a pill! Got indigestion? Pop a pill! Got insomnia? Pop a pill! And we are exposed to these messages from childhood.

The fact of the matter is our lives are hectic and making the kind of fundamental life-altering changes that could extend our life span, without drugs, seems like too much work, too much of an inconvenience or too hard to maintain. But the question is: what are the consequences of *not* making those changes? Don't we *want* to live to see our grandchildren graduate from university? Wouldn't we *love* to meditate on a mountaintop at 85? The answer is absolutely! So why do we often take yesterday's good intentions and throw them out the window today as if our mental, physical and spiritual health is something we can get around to later…when the kids are in school, when the kids are out of school, when we have more time, when we have more money, when we start our holidays…Start now! Make yourself a priority now!

Every minute we have in this life is a chance to start all over again. Isn't that great?

ASK YOURSELF...

- What signs and symptoms in my body am I ignoring (e. g. headache, poor sleep, constipation, heartburn, lack of energy, depression, neck pain, stress)?

- What kinds of self-sabotaging behaviors do I engage in that may cause disease in my life (e.g. overeating, lack of nutritious food in my diet, lack of exercise, excess weight, underweight, lack of sleep, too much stress, lack of life balance)?

YOUR WELLNESS STRATEGIES

- Take your journal and write a list of five things that your body is telling you (e.g. headaches, insomnia...). What do you think is causing these issues?

- Book a neuro-spinal scan and evaluation with your local Wellness Chiropractor to find out if your nervous system is working optimally.

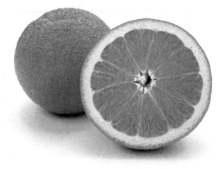

Chapter 2: Awareness – Be Aware And Awake In Your Life

– Andrée

"Only that day dawns to which we are awake"
    – Henry David Thoreau

Over the years in our respective practices, we have seen clients and patients stuck in negative patterns that affect their health and well-being in ways that hold them back from living a fabulous life. Even if those patterns were created decades ago, they continue to be repeated over and over again, as a matter of routine and through unconscious, mindless effort. Patterns are not inherently bad, however, patterns that keep you stuck or create negative or unwanted outcomes can be dangerous to your overall wellness. The sad part is that we sometimes don't even realize we are repeating patterns. Keep doing what you keep doing and you'll keep getting what you keep getting.

Many of us live our lives on autopilot, programmed like a computer. We repeat the same thoughts, conduct ourselves with the same behavior and perform the same tasks. It's the "hamster on a wheel" syndrome, stuck in a self-built cage, running in circles with no real purpose and with no end in sight.

Here's what this can look like…

- We have a job we don't particularly like but we show up every day and complain about our boss, the company, the hours they make us work, or the inadequate salary we receive;

- We feel down so we grab a chocolate bar hoping it will make us feel better – it happens regularly;

- We get home from work every night and we sit in front of the TV like zombies trying to forget our unfulfilling day at work, our financial problems or our relationship woes;

- Our relationship with our partner is strained but we put up with it because we don't want to rock the boat or we think to ourselves, "Oh well, it's good enough";

- We don't like our environment; the clutter, the weeds in the garden, the mess in our closets, but we tell ourselves we're too busy to do anything about it;

- We're often broke and complain to anyone who'll listen. We blame our partner who isn't good at saving money;

- We want desperately to lose weight but we don't. We complain that our clothes don't fit the way they used to, but every night we have a couple of chocolate chip cookies or cake or ice cream before going to bed. We don't exercise because it's just too much work and we feel too tired.

Do any of these scenarios sound familiar? Sometimes it takes a **S**ignificant **E**motional **E**vent (SEE) such as a heart attack, a divorce, or even the death of someone close to us to wake us up, rattle our cage, get us off that wheel and bring genuine awareness and attention to what we're doing to ourselves and to our lives.

When we go through an event that shakes us to the core of our foundation, we'll often feel the need to make changes. We become aware that the patterns we're repeating are not in our best interest, not giving us the quality of life that we want or deserve. But besides traumatic events that jolt us into a new reality, there are other instances in life that provide a more subtle wake-up call.

Being Awake and Aware in Your Life

What happens if you fall asleep at the wheel of your car? Well, if you're lucky you will slowly hit the gravel on the shoulder of the road and that will wake you up. If you're not so lucky, you could cross the line and hit an oncoming vehicle or head for the ditch or hit a tree…you get the point. Tragedy! Some of us are asleep at the wheel of our lives. We are swerving this way and that way; sometimes we hit the shoulder, maybe have a fender bender, catch a bad flu, or we lose intimacy with our partner. It shakes us so we wake up and make corrections or changes. But sometimes we cross that white line and tragically a relationship ends, we get seriously ill, we lose our job and we have to surmount incredible odds to regain control of our lives. All the signs that something was terribly wrong were there, but we either refused to see them or ignored them.

Maybe we experience a feeling of unrest, an unsettled feeling that something isn't quite right in our lives but we're not too sure what it is. We might be feeling uneasy, unhappy, lethargic or scattered, but we ignore it thinking that it is nothing and, anyway, we're just too busy to think about it. In both our practices, Dr. Nathalie and I have heard clients say they feel overwhelmed, apprehensive, sad, even disconnected. The good news is that people are noticing that something is wrong and are willing to voice it. It's a huge first step.

Being aware of what is going on inside our bodies and our minds is vital to living to our full potential. Awareness is really the first step to bringing about change in our lives so we can have a balanced and healthy lifestyle. So, what are the signs you could look for or be conscious of in order to become more aware of the changes you need make in your life? Here are a few thoughts to ponder:

- Do you find yourself snacking all the time and gaining weight? Perhaps you do this because you feel lonely, are lacking affection and, therefore, feeding your emotion?

- Do you feel tired or bored most of the time? Have you lost interest in hobbies or activities you used to like?

- Do you get angry or upset often even at insignificant things that would not normally set you off?

- How well are you sleeping? Do you wake up at all hours of the night and worry over a million things?

- Are you isolating yourself? Avoiding seeing friends or family?

These are just a few things, but I'm certain you could add to the list. What to do? The first step is truly becoming aware of the feelings. This means literally sitting down and coming into close contact with how you're feeling. This could mean writing in your journal about your feelings; taking time daily to reflect on what might be ailing you. You could also talk to a friend. Sometimes a trusted friend can shed much needed light on the issue. The idea is to give yourself permission to become aware of what is troubling you or what is making you feel not quite right.

Not everyone needs to go through significant emotional events in order to bring about changes in their lives. Some people can improve awareness simply by observing others' behaviors and actions in order to make necessary changes in their own lives. One thing is certain, awareness and acceptance of what is will bring on change. You need to know where you are and also know where you want to be in order to take the steps to get there.

Being aware means being present to yourself in every moment of every day! Notice how you react to events, how you feel around certain people, how you manage stressful environments and situations. Being aware means BEING rather than DOING! So many of us find it difficult to stop and just be. Awareness is composed of three elements: questioning, listening and feedback.

First, question how you're feeling; second, listen to your feelings and your thoughts; and, third, give yourself feedback on the patterns you're experiencing. For example, you notice that after a confrontation with someone you love, which left you feeling badly, the first thing you did was reach for a candy bar. STOP! Ask yourself, "Is this a pattern for me? Do I reach for food every time I feel bad?" Question other times when you reached for sugary or fatty snacks when you were feeling badly. You may discover a pattern in your actions. If so, what are you going to do?

Choices and Changes

Once you become aware of the patterns in your life that need changing, the next step will be to take ownership of these patterns. We are often faced with difficult choices in our lives. Changing some long-term patterns can be one of those. Some of the patterns we're stuck in have been with us for so long we can't begin to think how we might make changes.

Barbara's story may sound familiar to you. In the last few years of her marriage, Barbara felt terribly lonely and unhappy. At night sitting in front of the television, denying what was going on in her relationship, she would eat chips, chocolates, candies – you get the point. She was feeding her loneliness with junk food. Of course in no time at all she started putting on weight, her clothes didn't fit as well and when she looked in the mirror it only made her feel worse. It was a vicious cycle, she felt worse and then would reach out for some sweet snack that would give her that instant gratification but would make her feel awful later on. She was on that "hamster wheel" for three years. Not only was she unhappy, she subconsciously didn't like herself very much. On and on the pattern continued, until one day, she took a good look in the mirror while trying to get into a favorite dress, and her reflection said "STOP! What are you doing to yourself?"

Feeding her emotions was not only making her gain weight, it was affecting her self-esteem and was starting to affect her health. She was tired all the time, she lacked energy and just bending over to pick something up was difficult. It was a slow process, trying to undo the pattern and reconstruct the true Barbara.

Her first step was to visit a nutritionist, and change her eating habits by being conscious of what she was eating and when. She started noticing that whenever she was sad she would reach for unhealthy snacks. So, with the help of her coach she set some weight and exercise goals and got rid of all of the unhealthy foods in the house. Less temptation. In time, she got back to what I like to call her "fighting weight", the weight at which she felt good, energetic and attractive. It was all about choices. The choices you make need not be dramatic; you can start by taking baby steps, just one at a time.

What does it take to be awake in life? To help you along in discovering what you would like to change so that you can live a spectacular life, we have developed a few questions for you to work through, as well as provided some ideas for an action plan. Give yourself the opportunity to work with these questions and to develop your own plan. If you find this difficult, work with a friend or hire a coach. This is important! It's all about you!

ASK YOURSELF...

- If I could change one thing in my life right now, what would it be?

- Which areas of my life do I feel I've had to struggle with consistently? Here are some suggested areas, at which to look: your health, your relationships or your career.

YOUR WELLNESS STRATEGIES

- Decide on one action this week and change one thing that will have a positive impact on your life. Write down in your calendar or planner what day you intend to put your action into practice. Repeat this action for a period of four weeks, or until you believe you have established a new pattern. It takes 21 days to create a habit, so be patient with yourself.

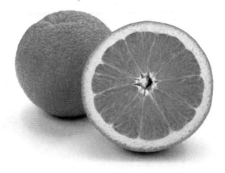

Chapter 3: Wellness: What Does It Mean?

– Dr. Nathalie

"Thousands and thousands of people have studied disease. Almost no one has studied health."

– Adelle Davis

How much energy do you want in your life? Do you want enough to play squash or go for power walks with friends during lunch? Do you want to have enough energy to play a game of tag with your kids after work or read them a story at bedtime? Do you want to spring out of bed every morning with tons of energy to make the most out of your day? How often do you just want to crash in front of the TV because you are too exhausted from your work day? The extent to which you feel healthy and well enough to keep springing out of bed is what this chapter is all about – your state of wellness. When people don't sleep well, don't eat properly, are depressed or anxious, something is wrong. Something is out of balance. Does this mean they're unhealthy? What do *you* think?

Wellness is an integral part of my everyday personal and professional existence. I was quite surprised at how difficult it was to find a definition for it in medical dictionaries. That said, "wellness" is a fairly new buzz word, while the word "health" has been used for centuries. This is why it was challenging to find a definition for wellness. Some of these dictionaries define health as a state of being well, sound or whole, in body, mind, or soul; and in particular, the state of being free from physical disease or pain. Because the use of the word wellness is so new, it's being used in a variety of contexts that concern me with some of its applications. While at an out-of-town conference, I overheard some people setting a time to meet at a bar for "wellness drinks". Wow! They certainly don't share my definition of wellness. Though, it could be a sign that the wellness industry is in the process of defining itself.

I think, as you may, that your well-being should be more than just about being disease or pain-free. I was, however, able to find some "non-medical" definitions of wellness. They describe wellness as a quality or state of being in good health, especially as an actively sought goal; or, as mental and physical soundness: physical well being, especially when maintained or achieved through good diet and regular exercise. And that definition sounds so much better to me! But my favorite definition comes from Dr. Patrick Gentempo, founder of the Creating Wellness™ Alliance. He is a true wellness pioneer who has defined wellness along with his team of health experts as:

"The degree to which an individual experiences health and vitality in any dimension of life – physical, biochemical and psychological"

The word "degree" implies that wellness and illness exist on a continuum. The human body is never static. Every decision you make moves you toward wellness or away from it. The question is which way are *you* moving? Dr. Patrick Gentempo further explains, "Health refers to biological function – blood pressure, body fat, etc. Wellness is a more expansive concept. It includes health and vitality. The Latin root *Vita* means life or that which pertains to the expression and experience of life. This is the power you have to live, grow and fulfill your maximum potential as a human being in the three dimensions."

When we talk about wellness, we are talking about how you experience your *entire* life, not just the number on the scale or the size of your clothes. Think about that for a second! You can have a fit, strong body that is free of disease and pain, and a mind that works like a steel trap. However, if you never smile or laugh, show compassion or give thanks, are you truly *living*? Are you truly well and balanced?

Stress is a fact of life and, believe it or not, we need stress to exist. Dr. Hans Selye, M.D., Ph.D., founder of the concept of stress, defined two types of stress. He named one Eustress (good stress) and the other Distress (bad stress). There will always be stressors in each of the three dimensions of our lives. We need to focus on the positive (good) stressors and try to minimize the negative (bad) stressors.

Examples of Stresses in the Physical Dimension

> Positive – exercise / digestion
> Negative – high blood pressure / insomnia

Examples of Stresses in the Biochemical Dimension

> Positive – drinking good, clean water / eating nutritious meals
> Negative – smoking / eating junk food

Examples of Stresses in the Psychological Dimension

> Positive – doing something you enjoy / accomplishing a goal
> Negative – financial worries / family strife

Unfortunately, it is possible to move toward wellness in one dimension and away from it in another. A friend of mine is a good example of that – she is a personal trainer who is in fantastic shape and eats really well. Her personal life is very stressful and she worries all the time, as a result, she only sleeps three hours a day and has for years. The fact that she can do three spinning classes in a row doesn't mean there should not be concerns for her health. You can't be good in two dimensions of your life and really bad in the other. There needs to be balance in all three dimensions, otherwise your body will eventually let you know. Also, keep in mind that stress is not just what happens to us, it is also how we choose to respond to events in our lives. We always have a choice!

As noted earlier, the human body is never static; wellness and illness exist on a continuum so every decision you make moves you toward wellness or away from it. The decision you made this morning to go to the gym moved you a little closer to wellness on that continuum. On the other hand, the fast food meal you ate last night moved you a little further away. Which way would you rather move?

The Disease Care Model

We need to start thinking differently about our health. Do we have a health care system or a disease care system? After all, when was the last time you went to the doctor because you were healthy?

Most people look at health from a Disease Care Model perspective. They look at health care as the detection and treatment of symptoms, disease and infirmity. That model looks mostly at a problem after it occurs. This is effective if you're in a car accident, for example, and need emergency surgery. However, does the system actually provide *true* health care? I believe it's a crisis care system and that it's mostly reactive. Although we are starting to see more public awareness campaigns for disease prevention, we all know how busy hospitals are these days. They are performing expensive and time-consuming tests on people who present themselves with potentially life-threatening symptoms, such as pain in the chest, trouble breathing or high blood pressure. What if we were to take some of the time and money that went into the diagnosis of an illness and put it toward a true lifestyle assessment? What are the risk factors that may have contributed to the problem? As it is now, the system is set up to manage symptoms and not their causes. There is simply no time to educate or empower patients to alter their lifestyles in order to create change. Again, it goes back to wanting the quick fix or the magic pill. Patients have been programmed to expect this approach and the medical system is doing its best to provide care. So, we have to start taking responsibility for educating ourselves! And then, with better educated patients, the medical system might actually begin to make the shift towards the Wellness Care Model.

The Wellness Care Model

The Wellness Care Model is something completely different and we all know how scary "different" can be. This model is based on promoting, regaining and/or maintaining health. The advantage of looking at our health from a wellness perspective is that we are able to look at the lifestyles that can lead to disease and, thereby, aim to prevent the disease from potentially developing. The Wellness Care Model is truly about caring for our health and identifying what we, as individuals, can do every single day to advance our own health and wellness.

I often give this example to my patients: an amazing medical procedure was able to detect that a man had a 75 percent coronary blockage. This great tool probably saved his life. But what about the lifestyle that led him there? What about the fact that he was 40 pounds overweight, never exercised, smoked and hated his job?! Did anyone ever address these issues with this patient? This is a great example of disease-care versus wellness-care.

Did you know that humans have the capacity to live well beyond 100 years? Yet the average life-expectancy for a North-American is around 76 years of age. Why knowingly cheat yourself out of a possible quarter century, when you might enjoy these extra years just by taking control of your wellness? You may, like many others, believe that your genes are largely responsible for your medical woes. A recent Yale study, however, showed that only 30 percent of health conditions (good and bad) are genetic-based. The other 70 percent are due to lifestyle. So let's stop blaming our genes and focus on what we can change – our lifestyle!

Be accountable for and to *yourself*. Change your life and learn to make better choices. *Stop* surviving and start thriving. Don't wait for something bad to happen before taking control of your well-being.

Measuring Your Wellness

How do you measure wellness? Is having a blood test going to tell you how "well" you are or is it just going to tell you how "not sick" you are?

Creating Wellness™ Centers use revolutionary technology to measure what is called your "Wellness Quotient" (WQ). Think of it as your wellness IQ. In comparison to a blood test that just tests for disease in your blood, the WQ measures your wellness based on a series of questions and tests related to the physical, biochemical and psychological dimensions of your life. This assessment will give you your quotient and also a report indicating what you're doing right in those dimensions and what you can improve upon! Creating Wellness™ has tools and strategies that can help you achieve increased wellness.

If you don't have access to a Creating Wellness™ assessment through your local chiropractic center, you may want to consider combining the services of a personal trainer, nutritionist, naturopath and life coach to help you measure and achieve your wellness potential. And again, if finances are an issue, try one of the above services as a start and consider the suggestions in this book.

As I always say to my patients, no one can be expected to make the optimum choices in all aspects of their lives at all times. There are, however, 365 days in a year – if you're moving in the right direction on the wellness continuum on most of those days, well, guess what? The momentum will keep you moving in the right direction.

Ask Yourself...

- What is my definition of wellness?

- Am I just surviving or thriving?

- What do I want more of for myself and what's stopping me (e.g. more energy, better sleep...)?

Your Wellness Strategies

- Make a list of your positive and negative stresses in the three dimensions of your life and figure out which way the scale is tipping and why.

- Make a list of three things that you can change in the next seven days and write down your strategy to get there in baby steps. Set yourself up for success!

- Find a Creating Wellness™ Center near you to discover what your Wellness Quotient is and create strategies to improve your WQ with the Creating Wellness™ System or create your own wellness team. To find the nearest Creating Wellness™ Center, visit www. creatingwellness.com.

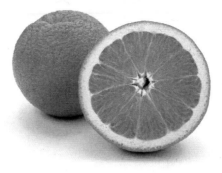

Chapter 4: A Clear Purpose

– Andrée

*"The meaning of life is whatever you ascribe it to be.
Being alive is the meaning. Follow your bliss and doors
will open where there were no doors before."*
— Joseph Campbell

Imagine yourself a year from now. Who do you see? What is your relationship like? Are you fit? What is your hobby? What job or career are you in? Are you excited to get out of bed in the morning, excited to start a new day? Are you able to see yourself in the future? Is it easy to see who you want to be, what you want to do and what you want to have by next year?

In my coaching practice, I have observed that eighty to ninety percent of people don't really know what they want in their career, in their relationships or in their life. When I ask my clients the questions, "What do you want?" or "What would make you happy?" I often hear, "I don't know, I just don't know." Why is that?

I do encounter people who do know what they want. I have had the opportunity to meet individuals who, for as long as they can remember, wanted to be a doctor, a lawyer, a musician or an athlete. Not all of us are that lucky. Not all of us grow up knowing our passion or our purpose. And what does that have to do with wellness, you ask? Everything! Living a life of purpose brings meaning, balance and happiness. If you know why you do what you do and you love doing it, there is a good chance that you feel good about yourself and feel successful and fulfilled.

Unfortunately, for many of us, we begin our adult life on autopilot. We graduate from college or university, land that first job and we feel pretty good! Life is good! We stay in that job, get promoted and move up the ladder. We get on our little hamster wheel, paying bills, buying stuff and then more stuff. We build our families, buy cars and 'toys' and keep running on that little hamster wheel.

We are so busy doing, doing, doing that we don't take time to think and reflect on what it is we really want in life. We let life happen to us instead of choosing what we want out of it. Some of us are stuck in the past, caught up in old patterns, unable to see a new way of being. And some of us are just afraid to dream, to imagine that we could have a better life. We lack the self-confidence to achieve our goals.

How can you find out what you really want in a relationship, in a career, for your health and your life in general? What I found in working with my clients and from talking with friends, is that it's much easier to first determine what you don't want. I asked a good friend what she wanted out of a relationship. She started listing all the things she didn't want in a relationship; she didn't want someone who smoked, she didn't want someone who was clingy, she didn't want a long distance relationship, and so on.

If we were to start the process by first deciding what we don't want, perhaps it would enable us to uncover and voice what we really do want. It may help to uncover a clear purpose and create a plan to get to where we want to go.

To help get you started, define what you want and clarify your purpose, I have developed a five-step process to help make it happen. It's not enough to just see it. You can visualize and dream all day long sitting on your couch and I can tell you from experience that it won't manifest. You need to get into action.

To start, you will need a journal or you can work on your computer. In your journal or computer program, create a table with five columns. See diagram 1 below;

1) In the first column, identify what you don't want/like;

2) In the next column, write what you do want or like, using your 'don't like' statements and stating them in a positive manner. For example one of your 'don't like' statements might be "I don't want to be fat."

Your "want" or "like" statement should read "I want to be at my ideal weight";

3) In the third column, write down why you want to be at your ideal weight. Is it because you want to feel healthy, or perhaps you want to feel sexier or maybe you want to run a marathon and be in top shape. Whatever your reason, write it down. This becomes your purpose;

4) Your next step will be to determine how you're going to reach your goal. This is where you develop your plan. Looking back at what you want and why, think of an action you can take today or this week to move you closer to your purpose;

5) The final step is your affirmation. This is a statement that confirms for you that you are not only committed to your action, but that you believe you are already there. You are engaging your mind at the subconscious level to succeed.

Diagram 1

What I don't want/don't like	What I want/like	Why do you want this – your purpose	What action can I take to be on purpose	Affirmation
I don't want to be overweight	I want to be at my optimum weight	I want to improve my health	I will go for a brisk walk today	I'm on my way! I enjoy feeling healthy and in control.

Your affirmations will anchor you to what really matters most to you – your dreams, your purpose.

This is the most exciting time of your life. Congratulations on giving yourself the gift of promise – a new way of living awaits you. What could be more exciting and promising than that?

Give yourself permission to dream and dream big. Spot opportunities to look at yourself differently – bolder, full of potential, the world wants you! Take small steps and start believing that the life you expect is within reach.

The momentum will come. Like a baby learning to walk, you'll be running in no time!

Ask Yourself...

Here are examples of questions you might ask yourself in order to develop your purpose and what you want in life. We recommend you start with one or two wants and set an action in place for each. This will help you recreate yourself one step at a time.

- What do you want more or less of? Do you want to be fit and at your optimal weight?
- Do you want to excel at a certain sport – maybe even teach it?
- Do you wish you were in a loving, romantic relationship?
- Would you like to have a new, fulfilling job?
- Would you like to have a better relationship with your friends, family and children?
- Would you like to learn a new skill or a new language?
- Would you like to have a more positive attitude?

Your Wellness Strategies

Once you've put words to your purpose and answered the "Ask Yourself..." questions, create a vision board. This fun exercise will help you carve out the dreams you want for your life. Do it with a friend – make it fun!

- Buy a stack of your favorite magazines. Cut out pictures that inspire you and glue them to a piece of Bristol Board. Everything on that board should be something you're going to strive to have or be within the next year.

- Make sure your vision board is somewhere where you see it regularly. I keep mine on the wall in front of my bed. I see it every morning when I wake up. It helps me focus on what is most important to me as I start my day. What a great way to start the day! Your mind will pick up the cues, consciously and subconsciously, and this can do wonders for helping you achieve your goals.

- Use the answers to your "Ask Yourself..." questions and create your own unique affirmation. Write your affirmation on a blank business card you can purchase at any office store and carry your card with you wherever you go – we call it "Affirmation on the Go!" Consider getting the card laminated – make it something that is meaningful to you. Take a peek at it whenever you need a little boost of motivation. Eventually, you'll memorize it and be able to recite it to yourself whenever you need to.

Enjoy the process. Make a game out of it. Have fun with it and may all your dreams come true.

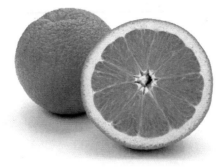

Chapter 5: Protein, Carbs And Fat – What Am I Eating?

– Dr. Nathalie

"Curious things, habits. People themselves never knew they had them."
– Agatha Christie

No book about wellness would be complete without addressing the overwhelming amount of information bombarding us every day about the food we eat. Good fat, bad fat, good cholesterol, bad cholesterol, low carb, high carb, low sugar, no sugar ... what and who to believe? Nutrition is a very complex and controversial topic. I believe that if you filled an Olympic stadium with nutritionists, dieticians and other health care professionals, the only thing they would probably all agree on is that vegetables are good for you!

There are so many variations on the theme of nutrition. Different diets recommend different types of foods, different combinations of food or different frequencies of eating. The truth is there is no one dietary plan that suits everyone. Our own body chemistry plays a huge role in whether we gain, lose or maintain weight. Have you ever wondered why Inuit people, who eat large quantities of fat and meat, have low rates of cardiovascular disease? Have you ever wondered why aboriginal people, who eat insects and berries, have great strength and fitness levels? Have you ever wondered why you can go on a cruise with your same-size best friend and eat the same food, yet you gain 10 pounds and she doesn't? Why?

The Metabolic Typing® Diet—A Different Way to Look at Your Diet

I came across The Metabolic Typing® Diet book by William Wolcott and Trish Fahey a while back and it made so much sense to me! Why do we try to eat the same diet when we are all so different? I knew, personally, that I felt so much better after eating certain foods while others seemed to rob me of my energy. I had instinctively narrowed down the food that gave me energy throughout the day and avoided the ones that seemed to slow me down! The concept of the Metabolic Typing® Diet is to create a diet that suits your individual nutritional needs. According to the authors, the long-term health benefits of a Metabolic Typing® Diet are:

- Natural weight loss without dieting or restricting calories

- Permanent weight loss without struggle, deprivation or hunger

- Achievement of your ideal weight, whether you are overweight or underweight

- Prevention of chronic disease

- Enhance immunity

- Improved resistance to cold, flu and recurrent infections

- Reversal of chronic or degenerative health disorders

- Slowing of the aging process

Metabolic Typing® takes into consideration parameters such as the following:

- Your autonomic nervous system – are you a sympathetic dominant or parasympathetic dominant (fight or flight)?

- Your carbo-oxidation rate – are you a fast oxidizer or a slow oxidizer?

- Your lipo-oxydative balance – are you more catabolic or anabolic?

- Your endocrine system (thyroid, adrenal, gonad and pituitary).

It may sound a little complex, but this information can be obtained quite easily through a proper evaluation. When your Metabolic Type® is determined, you then fall into three major categories: Protein Type, Carbohydrate Type and Mixed Type. Depending on your type, you will follow specific food guidelines as well as different suggested percentages of macronutrients. For example, a Protein Type might have suggested percentages of: 40 percent protein, 30 percent carbohydrates, and 30 percent fat, a Carbo Type might have percentages of: 25 percent protein, 60 percent carbohydrate, and 15 percent fat and a Mixed Type could have percentages of: 30 percent protein, 50 percent carbohydrate, and 20 percent fat.

Similar to the Metabolic Typing® concept is also Nutritional Typing™ which was developed by Dr. Joseph Mercola. The Nutritional Typing™ approach is similar to the Metabolic Typing® approach. It concentrates on the right food choices for your basic type—Protein, Carb and Mixed. For more information on either Metabolic Typing™ or Nutritional Typing™, you can visit www.metabolictyping.com or www.mercola.com.

As you can see, everyone has unique needs. My goal for this chapter is to give you the basic knowledge of the six types of nutrients in your diet. These nutrients perform different functions and together give your body the premium fuel it needs to work at its best. Keep in mind that the recommendations made in this chapter are general guidelines and do not necessarily take into consideration your Metabolic Type® or Nutritional Typing™.

Nutritional Basics: Energy Requirements

To start, you need to know what your energy requirements are. What does the word "calorie" really mean? A kilocalorie is the amount of energy it takes to raise the temperature of one kilogram of water one degree on the centigrade thermometer. We need a certain amount of calories to keep our body heated and running properly. Calories per gram are generic for the following:

Protein	4 calories per gram
Carbohydrate	4 calories per gram
Fat	9 calories per gram
Alcohol	7 calories per gram

Nutrients

Nutrients can be divided into two major groups:

1) Macronutrients – protein, carbohydrates and fat – which will be discussed in this chapter.

2) Micronutrients – vitamins, minerals and water – which will be discussed in other chapters.

Macronutrients – Protein

"I don't work out so I don't need a lot of protein!" If only I had a dime for every time I've heard my female patients say that! Proteins are an integral part of good nutrition and are absolutely essential, whether or not you are working out. We need protein in our diets to grow, maintain and repair every part of our bodies such as muscles, tendons, ligaments, skin, hair and nails.

Protein also plays a vital role in the formation of:

- Antibodies – needed for proper immune function
- Enzymes – required for the chemical processes of the body such as digestion
- Blood – red blood cells contain a protein called 'hemoglobin' that carries oxygen in the body
- Hormones – such as insulin, which regulates sugar and fat metabolism

Protein also provides the body with energy when we have lowered our intake of carbohydrates and fats, such as when we follow a low-calorie diet or do extreme physical activity.

Sources of Protein

Proteins are made up of 20 or so different amino acids. Eight of them are essential (the body can't make them on its own) and are required in our diet. Non-essential amino acids can be produced by our bodies from other amino-acids.

High quality protein: Protein that contains all essential amino acids in amounts that our bodies can use to build our own proteins such as meat, poultry, fish, eggs, and a good quality whey protein powder.

Lower quality protein: Protein that is missing one or more essential amino acid or has unbalanced amounts of amino acids such as legumes (beans, peas and lentils), nuts, seeds and grains (breads, pastas and cereals).

The World Health Organization and many national health agencies have independently conducted studies concluding that our daily protein requirement should be between 10 percent and 15 percent of our daily caloric intake. There is still much controversy over this and the percentages will vary from one source to another. In my opinion, protein percentages should take your Metabolic Typing® into consideration as well as your level of activity.

Daily protein considerations – basic guidelines by different levels of activity

Activity level	Protein per pound of body weight
Average adult	0.4 gram
Exerciser/active	0.5 to .75 gram
Athlete	0.6 to 0.9 gram
Bodybuilder	1.0 to 1.5 grams

If you don't have a food scale at home or if you are eating out in a restaurant, here is an easy way to "estimate" your protein content. One serving of protein, be it chicken, beef, fish or seafood, should be about the size of the palm of your hand – it will give you approximately 25 grams of protein.

Approximate Protein Content of Common Foods

- Egg (1 medium)..6 g
- Peanut butter , chunky (2TBSP) ....8 g
- Chick-peas, cooked (1/2 cup)......................................8 g
- Milk (8 oz.)...10 g
- Yogurt, low fat, plain (8 oz.)..12 g
- Almonds (1/2 cup)..15 g
- Tuna, fresh, cooked (3 oz.) ....23 g
- Ground Beef, lean, cooked (3 oz.)...............................24 g
- Chicken, boneless, cooked (3 oz.)...............................27 g

Try to get proteins and dairy from organic sources – grass-fed animals as opposed to grain-fed animals (see chapter #10 – "Is It Worth Going Organic?").

In my experience, female patients usually do not eat enough protein. These patients are having a hard time losing weight and are often frustrated. After reviewing their diet or looking at their Metabolic Type®, I often suggest an increase in their protein intake and a decrease in their carbohydrate intake. They often see great results! So instead of packing those low-fat carbohydrate snacks in our lunch bag, let's think about ways to load up on protein snacks instead. It might be difficult for vegetarians to increase their protein because they don't eat meat or for busy people with no time to cook. A quality whey protein powder can help give people the protein boost they need (see chapter #28 – "Whey" To Go!).

Don't be too tempted by protein bars as a quick alternative to other proteins because *most* bars also contain high levels of unwanted additives. Keep in mind that we can't live on protein bars alone. They should only be a last resort when fresh, wholesome foods are unavailable. Keep some in your bag for those times when you need something quick and handy (e.g., stuck in traffic or in a waiting room).

Macronutrients – Carbohydrates

Carbohydrates are the body's "high octane" fuel; their major role is to provide you with energy to think and to do. Carbs transform into glucose, which is carried through the blood to your brain, organs and tissues. If the body has enough energy, the glucose is stored as glycogen in the liver and in the muscles. When the body needs energy, it converts glycogen from the liver back into glucose. You need carbs to maintain those reserves and to prevent fatigue, dehydration and low energy levels. Adequate amounts of carbs also prevent our bodies from using protein for energy; which can leave the body weak and break down muscle.

There are two types of carbohydrates; simple and complex. Complex carbohydrates are higher in fiber and less refined than simple carbohydrate. Our carbohydrate intake should consist mostly of complex carbohydrates. While fruits are good for you, be aware that they fall in the "simple carb" category and need to be limited. The Canada Food Guide suggests between five and ten servings of fruits and vegetables per day, but your diet should focus more on vegetables than fruits.

Simple carbohydrates: found in fruits and juices, table sugar, corn syrup, honey, soft drinks and sweets.

Complex carbohydrates: found in grain products like breads, rice, cereals, pasta, beans and vegetable such as legumes.

To Carb or Not to Carb?

Carbs have gotten a bad rap over the years. What to believe? Even experts disagree. The scientific and medical community suggests that approximately 55 percent of your total daily energy intake should be provided via carbohydrates. Your carb and calorie intake depends on your activity level. If you sit at a computer all day and your best friend is training for a marathon, each of you will require a different number of carbs per day. But also, as explained previously, the Metabolic Typing® diet will determine your personal percentage of carbs. Until you find out your Metabolic Type®, here is a simple calculation. For example, if you want 55 percent of your energy to come from carbohydrates, you need about 275 grams of carbohydrates (based on a 2,000 calorie per day diet). Here's the math:

2,000 calories x 55 percent = 1,100
1,100 divided by 4 (4 calories per gram of carbohydrate) = 275 grams.

Approximate Carbohydrate Content of Common Foods

- Celery, raw (1 stalk)..1 g
- Broccoli, chopped raw (250 ml)......................................6 g
- Bread, whole wheat commercial (1 slice)....................16 g
- Apple with skin (medium)...19 g
- Banana 27g
- Potato, baked, skin (medium) ....34 g
- Plain bagel (10 cm diameter).......................................38 g
- Spaghetti, whole wheat, cooked (250ml).....................39 g
- Rice noodles, cooked (250 ml) ....46 g
- Brown rice, long grain, cooked (250 ml).....................48 g
- Muffin carrot commercial...49 g
- Apple crisp, homemade (250 ml)................................78 g

Years ago, western society went on the "no fat" bandwagon, and even though we are now eating less fat, the rate of obesity has increased. Simply put, we replaced fats with carbs. Consider that carbs in greater quantity than needed raise our insulin levels and are converted into fat. Add to that the poor quality of many available carbohydrate sources and it's a recipe for nutritional disaster.

Then we went on the "no carb" bandwagon. Some people were shocked at how much weight they lost in such a short amount of time; although a big part of it was probably water. But most people can't and shouldn't cut carbs out of their diet forever because the body needs them. For example, the brain needs a constant supply of carbs to function properly. When you begin to eat carbs again, your body will kick into survival mode and store them, worried that you'll deplete it of carbs in the future. Your metabolism will also slow down, further undermining your weight loss efforts.

A perfect example of the above is when I was preparing for my natural bodybuilding/figure competitions. My intake of carbs for weeks prior to the competition was as low as 40 grams/day. Within a week after a competition, when I reintroduced carbs to my diet, I would put on 10 pounds very quickly, even though my caloric intake wasn't much higher. As mentioned before, depriving our bodies of carbs compels us to store them as fat. In other words, your body goes into survival mode because it does not know when it's going to be fed next.

Glycemic Index

The Glycemic Index (GI) of a carbohydrate source is also an important factor to take into consideration. Entire books have been written on the subject and I will not attempt to go into great detail, but here is the "gist" of it. The Glycemic Index shows the various rates at which a carbohydrate breaks down and releases glucose into the blood stream. The faster the food breaks down, the higher the index. The Glycemic Index sets sugar at 100 and scores other food against that number, making it a great indicator of our body's insulin response. As a rule, insulin levels should be kept as steady as possible for optimal health. There is a ton of information available to you on the topic. You can go online and download lists of high and low Glycemic Index foods to guide you with your carbohydrate choices. The goal should be to choose more food from the low GI index to avoid a spike in your insulin levels. Insulin is an important hormone in regulating fat storage. Eating a low Glycemic Index diet promotes lower body fat and a leaner physique in the long term.

High levels of insulin could lead to unwanted stress on your pancreas and later lead to diabetes. Research shows that one out of three North Americans is now being diagnosed with Type 2 diabetes and 90 percent of those cases could be avoided with lifestyle changes. Insulin secretion can also have an impact on cancer development as it triggers the release of IGF (insulin growth factor) which stimulates cell growth. Therefore, it could potentially increase the number of cancerous cells. Insulin and IGF also promote inflammation in the body which can lead to other inflammatory diseases such as cancer, arthritis and heart disease.

Fiber

Fiber is important because it moves food through your digestive system, absorbing water and making elimination easier. Fiber also has a high satiety quality to it, so eating high-fiber foods will fill you up faster and you won't feel compelled to eat as much. The recommended daily intake of fiber is between 20 and 35 grams. Be aware that too much fiber may decrease your body's absorption of some vitamins and minerals. If you take a fiber supplement, do not take it at the same time as vitamins or prescription medication for this reason.

There are two types of essential fiber

Soluble fibers – They attract food but slow its passage in the small intestine where a lot of nutrients are absorbed. They have also been shown to decrease cholesterol levels and help control sugar levels.

Sources: oatmeal, oat bran, oats, corn bran, baked beans, lentils, and cereals.

Insoluble fibers – These fibers contribute to stool bulk because of their ability to trap water. They are commonly called "roughage".

Sources: Breads and cereals made from corn or wheat bran, fruits with seeds, broccoli, cauliflower, carrots, mushrooms and eggplant.

Macro-nutrients – Fat

Have you noticed that we are, as a population, eating less fat but are fatter than ever? How is that!? We need certain fats for our bodies to function properly. Fats are needed to help form cell membranes, carry fat-soluble vitamins, build tissue, produce hormones, protect vital organs, provide thermal insulation, transmit nerve impulses and, of course, provide fuel. Fats that are not produced by the body are called essential fatty acids (EFAs) and it means that they need to be acquired through diet (see chapter #12 – "The Power Of Omega-3"). But contrary to popular belief, we also need saturated fats. They form an important part of our body's cell membranes and eating mostly poly-unsaturated fats can have a detrimental effect on the chemistry of those cellular membranes. Read on…

The concept that fats are equally bad for you is outdated information. In their book, Eat Fat, Lose Fat, Dr. Mary Enig and Sally Fallon debunk certain facts about fat! Fat may not be the bad guy everyone paints it to be. Research is changing the way we look at fat. Fats that were once labelled "bad" may have some major health benefits after all. Supposedly "good" fats may not be as great as we once thought!

Types of Fat

Saturated fats

- Saturated fats are found mostly in meat and dairy products. They are also found in tropical oils like coconut and palm;

- Saturated fats are structured with their carbon bonds all occupied by hydrogen atoms making them highly stable;

- They are solid or semi-solid at room temperature;

- They are least likely to go rancid when heated and less likely to form dangerous free radicals.

Mono-unsaturated fats

- Mono-unsaturated fats are found in olives and olive oil, peanut oil, almond oil and canola oil*;

- Because of their chemical structures, they tend to be liquid at room temperature but become solid when refrigerated;

- They are relatively stable and do not go rancid easily with heat.

Poly-unsaturated fats

- Poly-unsaturated fat is found mostly in plant sources: safflower oil, sunflower oil, soy bean oil, corn oil, sesame oil, seeds and most nuts;

- Because of their chemical structures, they remain liquid at room temperature and when refrigerated;

- Omega-3 and Omega-6 are types of poly-unsaturated fats;

- Poly-unsaturated fats become highly reactive when subjected to heat and oxygen, leading to unwanted free radical formation.

---

* According to the Canola Council of Canada – Canola Quick Facts, today 80 percent of the acreage of canola is sown with genetically-modified canola.

Trans-fats

- They are produced by bombarding poly-unsaturated oils with hydrogen (hydrogenation) making them "resemble" saturated fats which makes them solid at room temperature and increases their shelf life;

- They are less expensive for the food industry to produce using cheap soy, canola or corn oil instead of the more expensive saturated fat sources;

- Trans-fats can be found in hardened margarines and shortenings, salad dressings, mayonnaise, cakes, cookies, crackers, fried foods and fast foods.

Best choices for cooking are saturated fats (coconut oil and palm oil) and fair choices are mono-unsaturated fats. Poly-unsaturated fats should never be used for cooking, as they are highly unstable when heated and lead to unwanted free radical formation.

Coconut Oil "Healthy" Facts:

- Coconut oil is 91.9 percent saturated fat – very stable for cooking;

- It's a high source of Lauric acid which has an effect on the immune system with antimicrobial properties;

- Coconut oil has been shown to increase thyroid activity because of its metabolic effect;

- The body can use coconut oil for energy, efficiently and quickly. Coconut fats are called medium chain fatty acids (MCFAs) and which normally don't get stored as fat. They are very helpful for weight loss;

- Most commercial coconut oils are not recommended because they are refined, bleached, and deodorized (RBD). Choose virgin coconut oil produced using low-tech and traditional processes.

There are some controversies among experts about the different types of fat. We have long been told that mono-unsaturated fats are the "best" fats, poly-unsaturated fats are the "acceptable" fats and saturated fats should be limited while trans-fats should be completely avoided. The authors of the book, Eat Fat, Lose Fat, are shedding a different light on fats and state that it is the free radicals from the extraction, processing and cooking of the poly-unsaturated fats, not the saturated fats themselves that can potentially initiate cancer and heart disease. This statement *should* change the way we consume fat. It is cutting edge information that, I believe, will soon become main-stream!

Your personal percentage of fat intake will differ depending on your Metabolic Type®, but as a guideline, here is a simple calculation. As an example, if you want 30 percent of your energy to come from fat, you need about 67 grams of fat (based on a 2,000 calorie per day diet). Here's the math:

2,000 calories x 30 percent = 600
600 divided by 9 (9 calories per gram of fat) = 67 grams.

Cholesterol

Although cholesterol has a bad connotation, it is important for our bodies as it is found in cell membranes, hormones, and is central to many body processes. There are two main types of cholesterol – Low Density Lypoprotein (LDL) cholesterol which has been called the 'bad' cholesterol and carries fat *to* body tissues and High Density Lypoprotein (HDL) which has been called the 'good' cholesterol and carries fat *away* from tissues. Health experts have recommended that we strive for lower levels of bad cholesterol and higher levels of good cholesterol. They also warn that if you have too much of the bad cholesterol in your body, it can potentially lead to heart disease. One little known fact is that cholesterol from diet has a limited influence on blood cholesterol levels. Our liver and cells create about 75 percent of our blood cholesterol level and only 25 percent comes from the food we eat.

There are some contradictions when it comes to cholesterol research. Some studies have shown cholesterol to be a great marker, while others point to the fact that there might be a higher death rate with normal or low cholesterol than high cholesterol. Research studies are uncovering the fact that it is *the oxidation of cholesterol* which may be causing heart disease. The "oxidized" or "damaged" cholesterol can lead to a complicated inflammatory process within the blood vessel leading to atherosclerosis plaque. There is, therefore, a need to also pay attention to inflammatory markers like C-Reactive Protein (CRP), serum amyloid A, white blood cell count and fibrinogen. Chronic inflammation is also a major cause of diseases like cancer, diabetes and arthritis. A popular choice for minimizing the risk of heart attacks by lowering cholesterol levels are statin drugs. However, like many other drugs, they have side effects and have been shown to decrease the heart critical nutrient – CoQ10.

Ask Yourself...

- Do I know how much protein, carbohydrates and fat I eat every day?

- Am I getting enough protein in my diet for my activity level?

- Do I know the difference between simple carbs or complex carbs?

- How much fiber do I have in my daily diet?

- Am I familiar with the Glycemic Index?

- Do I know which fats are good and which are not so good?

- Do I know which fats are preferable for cooking?

Your Wellness Strategies

- For the next three days write down your food intake – everything, no cheating!

- Calculate roughly the amount of protein, carbs and fat that you consume daily based on the above.

- How do you feel after eating certain foods, do you feel energized or tired and bloated?

- See a nutritionist or natural health practitioner for guidance on your eating habits.

- Consider a Metabolic Typing® Diet evaluation to determine your Metabolic Type®.

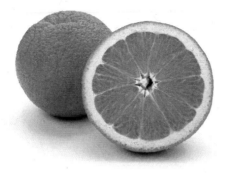

Chapter 6: Learning To Read Food Labels

– Dr. Nathalie

"We are indeed much more than what we eat, but what we eat can nevertheless help us to be much more than what we are."
– Adelle Davis

One of the best things you can do for yourself and your family is learn how to read labels on the food you buy. It takes a bit of extra time, but it's worth it. Knowing exactly what's in the food you're buying is an important step on the road to wellness. And thank goodness we have these labels. They only became law in North America a few years ago. Health Canada, for instance, introduced legislation to provide nutrition information on food labels in 2003. Labelling for most prepackaged foods became law in 2005 while small companies had until 2007 to introduce their nutrition labels.

Proper food labelling was a very positive step toward the promotion of healthier eating, but it is also very important to be able to interpret the labels and benefit from that information. Knowledge is power, but the application of knowledge is real power.

Since you can't just look at a packaged food item and tell whether it's healthy, you're going to need to do some reading. Let's look at a label and break it down:

1. *Serving size* – If you eat the serving size shown on the Nutrition Facts table, you will get the amount of calories and nutrients that

are listed. Always compare the serving size on the package to the amount you eat – we tend to eat much bigger portions than listed.

2. *Calories* – Calories tell you how much energy you get from one serving of the packaged food.

3. *Calories from fat* – The number of calories that come from the food's total fat count. If the number of calories from fat is close to the total number of calories, it means that the food you are eating is mostly fat.

4. *Percentage Daily Value (DV)* – The Percentage Daily Value given on a food label is based on the daily recommendations for key nutrients based on a 2,000 calorie diet. Depending on your body mass index (BMI) and daily energy output, you may need more or fewer calories. Anything below a five percent DV is considered low and above a 20 percent DV is considered high. It is important that you pay careful attention to the serving size when considering the daily value.

5. *Total Fat* – The combined saturated fats, mono-unsaturated fats, poly-unsaturated fats and trans-fats.

6. *Saturated Fat* – Saturated fat count has long been suggested to be kept low, but as discussed previously, not all saturated fats are as "bad" as once thought. Poly-unsaturated fats should also be monitored as they have been shown to be unstable when exposed to heat and oxygen – creating unwanted free radicals. For example, be aware of vegetable oils (see chapter #5 – "Protein, Carbs And Fat – What Am I Eating?").

7. *Trans Fat* – Should be avoided all together. They have been shown to raise cholesterol levels.

8. *Cholesterol* – Cholesterol has a bad rap but most people don't realize that the body manufactures most of our cholesterol; food adds only a small amount. The body needs a certain amount of cholesterol to function – our brain is partly composed of cholesterol! Concern yourself more with the type of fats you're eating.

9. *Sodium* – It's suggested not to consume more then 2,400 mg of salt per day. Be aware that processed foods tend to be very high in salt (e.g. frozen dinners and canned foods). Sodium ingredients

can be camouflaged in vegetables juices, soups and such. Words used: monosodium glutamate, baking powder, baking soda, disodium phosphate, sodium bisulfate, garlic/onion/celery salts and soy sauce.

10. *Total Carbohydrates* – This is the total amount of all sugar, starch and fiber in a food. What is more important here is the type of carbohydrate. Aim to consume complex carbohydrates and stay away from refined sugar. Refined sugars will show up on food labels under carbohydrates as "sugars".

11. *Fibers* – Any food with at least two grams or more per serving is good. The higher the fiber count the healthier the food likely is.

12. *Sugar* – Try to keep this number under five grams or less per serving, although there is no fixed recommendation for the total amount to eat per day. The sugar quantity listed on the label will include naturally occurring sugars (like those in fruit and milk) as well as those added. Check the ingredient list for specifics on added sugars. Fructose, glucose, lactose, galactose and maltose are not ones to be overly worried about in small amounts. Sugar ingredients to watch for: liquid sugar, invert sugar, liquid invert sugar, syrup, dextrose, dextrin, corn syrup solids, molasses, raisin syrup and sugar alcohols like isomalts, lactitol, mannitol, maltitol, sorbitol, xylitol. Over consumption of sugar alcohols can lead to bloating, diarrhea and flatulence.

13. *Protein* – A DV percentage is only required for protein if a product claims to be "high in protein" remember the amount of protein needed still varies from one person to another depending on level of activity.

14. *Vitamins and Minerals* – (vitamin A, calcium, vitamin C and iron). Calculations for vitamins and minerals are geared towards the prevention of deficiency/disease, not for the promotion of optimal body function. A high-quality multivitamin is strongly suggested to obtain optimal vitamin and mineral levels for your body.

15. *Reading the ingredients* – The ingredients are listed in order of quantity – largest to smallest. For example, try to stay away from food with high fructose corn syrup as the top ingredient.

Food Claims

"Reduced section" – When a food claims an ingredient is reduced it means it contains at least 25 percent less of a nutrient compared with a similar product (e.g. reduced calories, reduced salt, reduced cholesterol, etc.).

"Source of light section" – This means the food is associated with a significant amount of a nutrient. (e.g. fiber, vitamin C, etc.).

"Light" – This claim is only allowed on foods that are reduced in fat or reduced in calories. "Light" can also be used, however, to describe a feature of the food such as "light in color". If the word "light" is used on a food label, it must have a statement that explains what characteristic makes the food "light". There is one exception to this rule and it relates to sugar. "Light maple syrup" means "light in color" and does not need to have a statement with it. In this case, "light" does not mean low in sugar or calories!

Endorsements

How many times have you seen little symbols on packages of food that say this organization or that organization has given their endorsement claiming it's a "healthy" product? While their cause may be aligned with healthy eating and active lifestyles, these organizations are not always transparent about being paid to endorse a particular product. One of the risks we face as consumers, when we see such an endorsement, is over-doing it in terms of our consumption. Just because a product has been endorsed by a certain organization, does not mean we should eat the entire box in one sitting! Consumers must exercise due diligence when choosing these so-called "healthy" products.

ASK YOURSELF...

- How can I become more conscientious about what I'm buying?

- Do I routinely read grocery labels?

- Am I influenced by food packaging and/or endorsements?

Your Wellness Strategies

- Next time you go shopping, allow yourself time to read the labels.

- After reading the labels, see if you can make better choices with alternatives.

- Show your kids how to read labels too. Make it a game at the store. "Who can find the best option?"

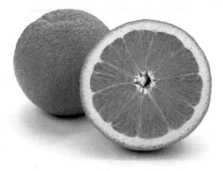

Chapter 7: Processed Foods – What Exactly Are We Eating?

– Dr. Nathalie

"Food is an important part of a balanced diet."
– Fran Lebowitz

What exactly is in the food you eat? Do you know? Because of stricter food labelling laws, most ingredients now have to be listed on food packaging. But how do you know what all those ingredients mean? How do you know if what you're eating is good for you? The fact is, most of the time we can't even pronounce the words on the ingredient list.

The best thing for us all is to eat fresh organic food that we prepare ourselves, but the reality is we don't always have access to fresh food and even when we do, it takes time to prepare fresh meals – time that we don't always have with our busy lifestyle!

We have become a fast food nation. Almost 90 percent of the money we spend on food is used to buy processed foods – 90 percent! Pop something in the microwave and voilà ... dinner is ready! But what are all those chemicals doing to our minds and our bodies? And what are the long-term repercussions for ourselves and our families of ingesting foods that have so many hidden calories, unhealthy fats and additives designed to chemically alter the food so it will taste better and last longer? If ever there was a strong statement against eating too much fast food it's the movie "Super Size Me" by Morgan Spurlock. It's the true story of a man who eats nothing but McDonalds for 30 days. Everyone should watch this movie with their family; it really is an eye-opener as to what junk food can do to your body.

In researching this book, I found an incredibly disturbing statistic from the United States Food and Drug Administration (FDA): the FDA currently lists approximately 2,800 international food additives and about 3,000 chemicals which are deliberately (and legally) added to our food supply. When you consider the number of chemicals used to grow and process food, it is possible that we will consume between 10,000 and 15,000 chemicals a day by the time our food reaches our stomach. Just pause for a moment and really think about that. Ask yourself, "Is that the kind of thing you really want to be feeding your family?"

Now, we all know that manufacturers use food additives to make food taste better and last longer – color, flavor, texture, stability, enhanced nutrient composition, and resistance to spoilage are just some of the characteristics that additives give our food.

Before you reach for your next package of processed food, you might want to familiarize yourself with these definitions – some of them may change your mind.

- *Anti-microbial agents* – preservatives that prevent spoilage and inhibit the growth of microbes such as bacteria, fungi, and viruses. Less harmful examples include acetic acid (vinegar) and sodium chloride (salt), but nitrates and nitrites are also used to preserve foods. The problem is, these anti-microbial agents may be creating super bugs, which are learning to procreate in ways that are resistant to anti-microbial agents and rendering us sick as our bodies have not learned to deal with them.

- *Antioxidants* – preservatives that prevent rancidity of fats in foods and other damage to food caused by oxygen. Some examples of preservatives are ascorbic acid (vitamin C), and tocopherols (vitamin E). While these vitamins can be used by our bodies, the synthetic kind or those derived from genetically-modified foods are not recommended because of their potential dangerous health effects.

- *Artificial colors* – food coloring is added to foods to enhance its appearance. Food colors are a mix of vegetable dyes and synthetic dyes approved by the FDA for use in foods. Some of these were primarily deemed safe and then later de-listed; others are still being studied. Some have already been linked to ADD and ADHD in children.

- *Artificial flavors, flavor enhancers* – chemicals that mimic natural flavors. They are just that, "chemicals".

- *Bleaching agents* – substances used to whiten foods such as flour and cheese, such as peroxides. Chemicals again!

- *Nutrient additives* – vitamins and minerals added to improve nutritive value. Most often these are derived from genetically modified foods. It's much better to get your nutrients from real, wholesome foods.

- *Thickening and stabilizing agents* – ingredients that maintain emulsions, foams or suspensions or lend a desirable thick consistency to foods. More chemicals.

The FDA decides what additives can legally be added to foods. To obtain permission to use a new additive, a manufacturer must test the additive and satisfy the FDA that it is effective (it does what it is supposed to do) and can be detected and measured in the final food product. Then the manufacturer must study the effects of the additive when fed in large doses to animals under strictly controlled conditions to prove it is safe for consumption. It is important to note that while the FDA has the final say in what is approved, it is the manufacturers (the ones who will make money by selling the product) who provide the evidence for the safety of the additives. Does that sound right to you?

Beyond the chemicals and additives approved by the FDA, which must be listed in the ingredients list, there is also a list known as the GRAS (Generally Recognized as Safe) list. These are some 700 substances which are exempt from complying with the above approval procedure because they have been used for such a long time and have no *known* hazard. These items are not required to be put on an ingredient label. Instead, all that is required are the words "artificial flavor" or "artificial coloring" or "natural." Just because something has been used for a long time and is considered *generally* safe, does that mean we should consume it? Why take the chance?

Particularly Problematic Dyes and Additives

Synthetic food dyes are used to color our food. Use and regulation differ from one country to the other. The FDA has recently been petitioned to ban eight artificial dyes: two yellow (Tartrazine and Sunset Yellow FCF), two reds (Erythosine and Allura Red), two blues (Brilliant Blue FCF and Indogotine) and Fast Green FCF and Orange B. Other more natural alternatives are currently in use in some European countries. North American companies need to follow suit.

Tartrazine (yellow number 5) – this food coloring can cause an allergic reaction in some people – about 1 in 10,000. Symptoms include hives, itching and nasal congestion, sometimes severe enough to require medical attention. There is a reported link between Attention Deficit Hyperactive Disorder (ADHD) in children and the use of this food coloring. The law requires that tartrazine be listed on all labels of food that contain it.

MSG (monosodium glutate) – is used widely in restaurants, especially Asian restaurants. MSG provides a basic taste called 'umami', which gives food a meaty taste. In some people, MSG produces an adverse reaction called the 'MSG symptom complex'. Symptoms of this include burning or sensation in the chest, facial flushing, and throbbing headaches. MSG has also been linked to eye problems, fatigue, disorientation and depression. Meals containing carbohydrates seem less likely to induce these adverse effects than meals with broth. Despite this, MSG has been deemed safe for consumption but it is kept out of foods for infants because very large doses have been shown to destroy brain cells in developing mice. MSG is used as a flavor enhancer in countless processed foods. But while it works to enhance your food's flavors, it is also at work doing potential damage to your brain and body. It's hard to know how much MSG you're eating because it has many different names. Choosing fresh, unprocessed foods is your best bet or trying to become familiar with the hidden names for MSG. To find out more about the different aliases of MSG and which foods contain it log on to: www.msgmyth.com.

Food Dyes

There is a wealth of information out there on additives, so it's important to do your homework. You can also contact your local health department to find out what information they might have on food additives. Taking a few hours now could add years to your life down the road.

Health Effects of Eating Too Many Processed Foods

With all of the many chemicals and additives that we ingest each day through processed foods, there has been growing concern over their health impact on North Americans. Some of the major health concerns include:

Obesity – obesity rates and the health risks associated with obesity have skyrocketed over the last 20 years. A recent study compared caloric intake in children on days when they ate in fast-food restaurants to days when they did not. They soaked up 126 calories more on fast-food days, which could translate into weight gain of 13 pounds per year due to fast food alone. The increasing rates of obesity associated with diets high in processed foods also lead to many serious illnesses including heart disease, stroke, diabetes and cancer.

Diabetes – Processed foods generally have a much higher sugar content than fresh foods like fruits and vegetables. They also contain types of sugars that break down quickly, providing a rush of glucose throughout the body. Too much glucose accumulation puts stress on the pancreas, which can lead to diabetes.

Heart Disease – Many processed foods contain trans-fats and other unhealthy fats which can lead to an increase in the risk of heart attack and stroke. Processed foods are also very high in salt. Diets high in salt are often associated with an increased risk of heart disease. For instance, one half cup of a popular canned chicken noodle soup has 37 percent of the daily recommended amount of sodium.

Cancer – A study involving 400 Canadian men between 50 and 80 years old found that those who ate a diet high in processed foods including processed meats, red meats, organ meats, refined grains, white breads and soft drinks, had a 2.5 percent increased risk of prostate cancer. Several other studies have shown links between processed foods and increased rates of breast and colorectal cancers.

Ask Yourself...

- Do I pay attention to the foods I eat?

- Do I eat junk food when I am in a hurry?

- Am I eating nutritional foods that will give me energy (wholesome foods)?

- Am I teaching my children good eating habits?

Your Wellness Strategies

- Next time you do your groceries try to spend more time in the outer perimeter of the store, the fresh food aisles. There, you will find fresh vegetables, fish, chicken and meats. Generally, middle aisles contain processed foods. For a week, see if you can feed yourself and your family with food purchased from the outer aisles of the store.

- Count how many times you eat processed foods in one day. Pick one or two of those foods and eliminate them for one week.

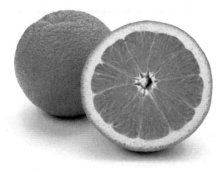

Chapter 8: Food For Your Heart And Soul

– Andrée

*"With every experience, you alone are painting your own canvas,
thought by thought, choice by choice".*
– Oprah Winfrey

So now that we've learned a bit about why it's so important to feed your body the right foods and the right nutrients, it's time to take a look at another area that needs just as much attention and tender loving care – your spirit. What are you feeding your heart and soul?

Your heart and soul – the spiritual you – needs to be fed as well. After all, we are not complete without mind, body and soul working as one. When one works harder than the other, we create an imbalance; imbalance can create unease, stress and ultimately disease. We could have the most beautiful bodies ever, cut like gods or goddesses, but if our hearts and souls are wanting, can we truly be happy? If not, we could be heading towards some serious side effects such as stress, emotional or mental breakdown, or even disease.

Much like a computer, our inner selves – our hearts, our souls, our spirits – have an operating system. This operating system was created over many years, with a lot of input from our parents, siblings, friends, teachers, and other people of influence around us. This system is what makes us do the things we do – good, bad or indifferent. Sometimes when we live and work on autopilot, those earlier inputs make key decisions in our lives and we're not even aware they're being made! And because the inputs are so ingrained in us, we think that is how life ought to be lived – by doing the same things the same way, over and over again, using the same set of criteria and judgments we have always used. Sometimes, however, something wonderful happens and we wake up; we tune into the signs around us and we want to change and grow.

All of us have coasted at one time or another in our lives because we were simply unaware of the damaging patterns that drove our behavior, or we simply weren't ready to confront them. Think about your childhood, for example. Were you surrounded by negativity and criticism? If so, you may tend to engage in negative, critical thinking almost automatically. As a result, you may also look for similar negative patterns in people and situations because it's your known mode of operation. You may even be addicted to creating negative, critical situations in order to keep your robotic state functioning subconsciously.

Eventually, however, all of that "stuff" that you have so mindlessly been inputting into your operating system, much like a computer, goes unfiltered and you catch a virus, or get sick, or angry or depressed or anxious. And when your spirit, or computer, is contaminated, it slows down. It can't handle even the simplest of tasks so it corrupts files (or thoughts) and eventually stops working altogether. The key is to clean out the garbage, clear out your hard drive and rebuild a functioning operating system with quality input.

Today, you have taken an important first step towards becoming positive and affirming towards yourself, and becoming more aware of the ways you might be contaminating your heart and soul. You are reading this book. Good for you! What else are you feeding your heart and soul with? Take inventory of the books you read, the magazines you purchase. Does what you read make you feel good about yourself or make you compare yourself to others? Does your reading material encourage a healthy lifestyle, or suggest unhealthy behaviors such as crash diets or various potions and lotions to improve your appearance?

We are often "force-fed" unhealthy ideas about who we should be, what we should be and what we should look like. Discerning from the myriad of information that is out there is not always easy, but once again, the number one key to finding what is good and not so good for you is awareness.

Once armed with information, you can make better, educated decisions about what you feed your heart and soul.

The saying "Buyer Beware" has never been truer. Be aware of what you read and what you listen to. Be aware of what you put into your heart and soul in the way of information, whether it's from media or from well-meaning people around you. Check in with how the information is making you "feel". If any of the information you are reading, viewing or listening to gives you a feeling of unease or a feeling that you are not measuring up, please do yourself a favor, and verify the source – even if the information is coming from a well-meaning friend. Always, always check in with your internal self, your intuition, to see if these are the right choices for you. Take TV, for example. It bombards us with negative news all day long. You may be desensitized to it and may not notice its effects, but subconsciously your mind will have these images playing over and over again!

To feed your heart and soul the nutrients they need, hang out with positive people who have awareness and are building healthy lives for themselves. Find a hobby that makes your heart sing – join a choir or take an exotic cooking or dancing class. Other heart and soul foods can include watching an uplifting movie, listening to a motivational CD, meditating, or reading positive affirmations. Whatever it is, find something that really energizes you, something that feeds your spirit. There are so many choices and options for you to choose from, choose one that uniquely satisfies you.

Ask Yourself...

- What am I feeding my heart and soul, my inner self?

- What changes should I make to my daily heart and soul diet?

- What would I have more of if I were to let go of my internal negativity?

- What type of music boosts me and makes me feel good?

- Am I listening to mindless TV and negative news?

YOUR WELLNESS STRATEGIES

- Take five to ten minutes every day this week to meditate and reflect.

- Write down all the things you are grateful for in your journal and refer back to them when need be.

- This week, write down one action in your journal that you can take to add positive ingredients to your heart and soul diet.

- Stop listening to the radio's bad news – snowstorms, accidents and traffic jams.

- Listen to educational, inspirational and motivational CDs.

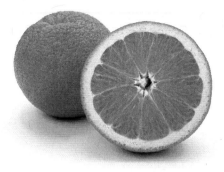

Chapter 9: Less Is So Much More!

– Andrée

"Go confidently in the direction of your dreams! Live the life you've imagined. As you simplify your life, the laws of the universe will be simpler."
– Henry David Thoreau

As we mature, we may find ourselves wanting to simplify our lives. We may want to de-clutter, downsize, rid ourselves of useless things, stop running around and so on. We may take a closer look at what's in the fridge and on our kitchen shelves, possibly because we have accumulated pots of jelly on those shelves and our hips and belly. It's a real wake-up call to realize that all of this extra stuff is not only unnecessary, it's actually detrimental to our well-being.

Once we begin to realize that racing around and accumulating "stuff" may not be the key to eternal happiness after all, we'll probably find ourselves wanting to make some changes. At a subconscious level, we already know what needs to change but accepting those changes takes time and understanding.

Simplicity in life is really about letting go. It's about peace of mind, about being happy with what and who we are and what we have. It doesn't mean we stop wanting things, but it does mean that we start wanting the *right* things to really fulfill ourselves in all aspects of our lives.

Simplicity in Food

In its purest form, simplicity in life is about feeling well in all areas of our lives. Eating well, for example, can be simple, fun and nurturing for our bodies. As suggested by Dr. Nathalie, including organic fruits, vegetables, meats and nuts in your daily meal plan should not be made complicated. Look for fun and healthy recipes that you can prepare ahead of time to make your evening meals quick and easy, without the fuss of preparation after a long day of work.

Take time to clear your fridge and cupboards of processed foods and any high sugar/high simple carbohydrate food items; the process itself will make you feel lighter. Without the temptation of sweets to snack on in the evening, you will be well on your way to a healthier you. Also be sure only to have the food you need in your kitchen; you'll have less clutter and fresher food choices.

Simplicity in Your Home and Surroundings

Establishing simplicity in your life can take a little time in the beginning, but it will ultimately save you time and energy and promote well-being in the long run.

Food for Thought...

- Do I have clothes in my closet that I haven't worn for one year or more? Why am I hanging on to them? Wouldn't they better serve the needy?

- Do I have files dating back more than 10 years?

- Do I have boxes in my storage space or basement with unknown content?

- Do I have stacks of magazines all over my coffee table or piles of envelopes and bills on the dining room furniture?

When you look around your house, do you get a sense of simplicity and airiness or a sense of clutter? The clutter around you can give you a feeling of being stuck, being tied down and even suffocated. Imagine those times when you're trying to find that one piece of paper with an important phone number, but it's lost in the stack of papers and bills on your desk. The stress is incredible and it's anything but simple. Being able to find what you're looking for in a few minutes, rather than a few hours, will not only reduce some stress in your life but also give you more time to enjoy leisure activities. Simplicity is freedom. So go ahead, re-organize your closet, your desktop, your files and simplify your life.

Simplicity in Your Leisure Activities

Ensuring you're feeling well is also a simple act of promoting your well-being – like going for a walk alone, with someone you love or with your puppy! A brisk 30-minute walk every day is a good aerobic exercise, good for your heart and good for your emotional and mental well-being.

If you're having a stressful day at work, go for a walk at lunch and notice how your mood changes. Leisure activities need not be complicated. You can watch a good movie, read a great book, or do something more interactive like attending an exciting and positive workshop. Take a moment to smell the roses in life...literally!

In springtime, walk through a greenhouse, see all the new blossoming flowers, shrubs and trees and take all the beauty in. It's a simple and pleasant activity that can bring a smile to your heart. Give yourself permission to do it. So many pleasures can be derived from very simple things.

Simplicity in All Things

Simplicity also entails some *nots*. That means *not* worrying, *not* stressing and just going with the flow. Are you a drama queen? Any small event can become a major catastrophe when you're one of these. Example: It's Sunday afternoon, you go to the ATM and when you try to withdraw money the machine tells you that you are overdrawn. You panic. You're frantic. "Oh my gosh, what happened?" you say out loud. Then you think, "What if it's identity theft?" You start to experience shortness of breath, your pulse races, you start thinking that you'll have to cancel all your credit cards and on and on.

But what if you were to take a step back and let go of that drama? What if, in that moment, you consoled yourself and rationalized that you'd check with the bank first thing the next morning because there must be a perfectly good explanation for the lack of funds in your account? The fact is, the second response will not only calm you but is a more appropriate reaction under such circumstances and will allow you to think clearly about your options. The drama isn't necessary and it certainly won't benefit you.

Legitimate stressful events do happen, but sometimes we create them for ourselves. Simplifying our thoughts and stepping back to assess such events does wonders for our well-being. Try to look at events in your life without getting involved in the drama of it all and going into panic mode. What a difference it can make.

Simplicity means keeping a positive attitude, smiling more often, and looking for the good in things, people and events. When you introduce simplicity to your lifestyle, you'll see how it brings you peace of mind. Having a well-organized, simple life will at the very least reduce our stress level, which in turn will lead to better sleep patterns, better relaxation and give us the head space to make better choices in our lives. In short, simplicity will give a boost to our overall wellness.

ASK YOURSELF...

- What does simplicity mean to me?
- What makes me happy or gives me peace of mind?
- Which area of my life needs the most simplifying?
- What could I do without?
- Where can I simplify right now?

YOUR WELLNESS STRATEGIES

- Simplify one thing this week in one facet of your life – will it involve your home environment, work, a relationship or your body?
- Choose one thing to simplify every week for the next 12 weeks and watch your life change.

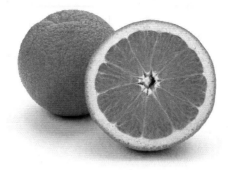

Chapter 10: Is It Worth Going Organic?

– Dr. Nathalie

"Turbulence is life force. It is opportunity. Let's love turbulence and use it for change."

– Ramsay Clark

Over the years, a number of questions related to organic foods and products have been raised by my patients. Their questions range from, "Is the food I'm buying really organic?" to "Is organic food worth all the fuss?" I wanted to be able to answer their questions. So I started doing some research on the subject in order to have a solid understanding of the various opinions out there. It is also important, as with many of the topics covered in this book, to consider the merits of the information sources – who and what to believe?

Have you ever noticed that the fruits and vegetables in the organic section of the grocery store are often more expensive and sometimes not very appetizing? Do you ever think: Why should I pay more for something that visually pales in comparison to its nice, shiny and much bigger conventional counterpart?

In the past decade, U.S. organic sales have grown at least 20 percent each year. In 2004, organic food and beverage sales topped $15 billion and sales are projected to more than double by 2009.

The Real Organic

Organic certification is a detailed process for organic food producers and includes standards that stretch above and beyond standard government regulations that apply to non-organic producers. Requirements vary from country to country, but generally involve a set of production standards for growing, storage, processing, packaging and shipping.

Organic standards can, and generally do, include:

- Avoidance of most synthetic chemicals – fertilizers, pesticides, antibiotics and food additives;

- No use of genetically-modified organisms;

- Production on farmland that has been free from chemicals for at least three years;

- Random and periodic on-site inspections.

Conventional Farmers Use	Organic Farmers Substitute
Chemical fertilizer	Natural fertilizer
Insecticides	Insect predators and barriers
Synthetic herbicides	Crop rotation, tillage, hand weeding, cover crops and mulches

Take note that your local farmer's market can be a great source of fresh products even if they are not certified organic. The food will be fresh and locally grown and will, therefore, not have been subject to a lengthy transport schedule. You'll feel good about supporting your community, as well as taking part in reducing transportation pollution.

Canadian Organic

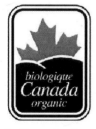

In Canada, the government has published a national organic standard, but as a guideline only – legislation is still in the works. Organic certification is, however, provided by private sector organizations and is identifiable by the logo. The logo is a part of new *Organic Products Regulations* announced in December 2006 and will tell you whether you are purchasing products that are federally certified as organic. Following the phase-in period that ended in December 2008, it will be mandatory for all organic products to be certified for interprovincial and international trade.

U.S. Organic

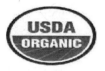

U.S. regulations divide organic labelling into four categories:

1. 100 percent organic – products must contain only organic ingredients;

2. Organic – products must be at least 95 percent organic by weight;

3. Made with organic ingredients – processed products that contain at least 70 percent organic ingredients;

4. Processed products with less than 70 percent organic ingredients may list ingredients on the information panel but not on the front of the package.

In the U.S., organic certification is recognizable with this label – the seal may appear on products in the first two categories only.

International Organic

Because of the great demand and the limited capacity of local farmers, organic foods are being imported from countries like China, Sierra Leone and Brazil, where standards are difficult to monitor.

Internationally, organic equivalency negotiations are underway to establish some kind of organic standard from country to country. International councils are also being created to monitor the standards including the International Federation of Organic Agriculture Movements (IFOAM), the Organic Crop Improvement Association (OCIA) and Ecocert. It's a work in progess and not all countries have the same standards, so exportation can be a grey area at this point.

The Organic Dietary Debate

Pesticides

Whether pesticides are harmful to humans is still a leading debate in the produce world. Because of pesticides, the average farm land yields 200 percent more than it did before they were introduced 70 years ago; quite an incentive for some people to ignore the potential health hazards.

The Environmental Protection Agency (EPA) however, considers 60 percent of herbicides, 90 percent of fungicides and 30 percent of insecticides to be carcinogenic. Pesticides have been shown to have many negative effects on our health like: neurotoxicity, disruption of our endocrine system, and immune system suppression.

The following foods tend to be most contaminated and should be bought organic as often as possible:

Fruit:

- Apples
- Cherries
- Grapes
- Nectarines

- Strawberries
- Peaches
- Pears
- Raspberries

Vegetables:

- Celery
- Cucumbers
- Green beans
- Lettuce
- Peppers

- Potatoes
- Pumpkins
- Spinach
- Squash

The following foods tend to be least contaminated:

Fruit:

- Bananas
- Blueberries
- Grapefruit
- Kiwis
- Mangoes
- Melons

- Oranges
- Papayas
- Pineapples
- Plums
- Tangerines
- Watermelon

Vegetables:

- Asparagus
- Avocados
- Broccoli
- Cabbage
- Cauliflower
- Eggplant
- Onions
- Peas
- Radishes
- Tomatoes

Genetically Modified Foods

Genetically modified foods only began hitting grocery shelves in 1995. Now, a whopping 90 percent of an average person's grocery budget in the western world is spent on processed foods and 70 percent of that food has been genetically modified in some way or another. Hybrid varieties of genetically modified fruit are often appealing because they're seedless and they taste sweeter than conventional kinds; but be aware that they also contain a lot more sugar.

To spot a genetically modified fruit or vegetable, look at the little sticker that shows the 'PLU code'.

- The PLU code for a conventionally grown fruit consists of four numbers – i.e. 1022
- The PLU code for an organically grown fruit is five numbers beginning by the number 9 – i.e. 91022
- The PLU code for a genetically modified fruit is five numbers beginning by the number 8 – i.e. 81022

Hormones

Over the past two decades chickens have grown 25 percent bigger in less time and on less food, while the average cow produces 60 percent more milk, all due to synthetic hormones. Producers reap big, but the cost to our health is questionable.

Antibiotics

Antibiotics, which are put in animal feed and are present in non-organic animal products, increase antibacterial resistance in humans, creating "super bugs" and major health concerns in the long term.

Nutrients

Besides being pesticide-free, hormone-free, and antibiotic-free, another health benefit of organic food is that it tends to have more nutrients than conventional produce.

> *"On average, conventional produce has only 83 percent of the nutrients of organic produce. Studies have found significantly higher levels of nutrients such as vitamin C, iron, magnesium and phosphorus, and significantly less nitrates (a toxin) in organic crops."*

– Mercola.com

Other Reasons to Go Organic

- Organic food tastes great!
- Organic farms respect water resources
- Organic farmers build healthy soil
- Organic farmers work in harmony with nature
- Organic farming helps keep rural communities healthy
- Organic farming slows down the depletion of nutrients in the soil

When to Really Choose Organic

- When buying fruits and vegetables that have high pesticide levels – see previous list;
- When buying meat, poultry, eggs and dairy; buying organic items greatly minimizes exposure to toxins, hormones and antibiotics. Look for meat from grass-fed animals. If the animals have been fed organic corn or soy, their meat and eggs will remain high in pro-inflammatory Omega-6 and low in Omega-3 (see chapter #12 – "The Power Of Omega-3");
- When buying baby food; a 1995 U.S. study found more than 16 pesticides in about half of the non-organic baby food tested. Chemicals even in small quantities have a big impact on such tiny, growing bodies.

When Organic Doesn't Mean As Much

- Buying seafood, whether caught in the wild or farmed; it can be labelled organic even if mercury and chemical compounds are present;

- Buying cosmetic products; although everything you put on your body is absorbed through your skin, due to lax laws, any cosmetic product can call itself natural but still be synthetic. To evaluate the products that you're using, log on to www.ewg.org (see chapter #34 – "Cosmetics – Painting A Different Picture");

- Organic milk; better than non-organic milk as it will be pesticide-, hormone-, and antibiotic-free but pasteurization can be of concern. The process of pasteurization destroys the good enzymes, reduces vitamins, dramatically reduces protein content, and is associated with allergies, increased tooth decay, colic in infants, growth problems in children, osteoporosis, arthritis, heart disease and cancer. Clean raw milk may be an alternative. Visit www.rawmilk.com to learn more about it. At the time of writing, raw milk is not available in Canada;

- Organic grains, like regular grains, are metabolized to sugar. So, even if you are purchasing organic whole grain bread, for example, it may still disrupt insulin levels if taken in quantity;

- Sugar is sugar even if it's organic. It is not the best choice to make for your health regardless of the organic label! So again, don't be fooled by great marketing strategies trying to sell you "organic" if, essentially, the food is not good for you in the first place.

There is no doubt that eating organic is better, but if you don't have access to organic or if it's too expensive, it's still better to eat conventional vegetables and fruit rather than to avoid them altogether.

Do Your Best!

You might be thinking that going organic is too much work, that you don't have the resources, the time or the money. Indeed, healthy eating is a commitment, but eating organic food is not only better for you, the way it tastes and the way it will make you feel will have you converted in no time. Hopefully, with the demand of organic foods skyrocketing, getting these foods will become easier and less expensive over time. Just do your best, start changing the way you eat slowly and feel good about it! There are now a growing number of organic food services that will deliver to your door! "Ding dong! Your fresh organic food is here..."

Organic Resources

The following sites can help you in your quest for organic foods. There are a multitude of other good resources online:

- Local Harvest
  www.localharvest.org

- Eat Well Guide: Wholesome Food from Healthy Animals
  www.eatwellguide.org

- Food Routes
  www.foodroutes.org

- Community Involved in Sustaining Agriculture (CISA)
  www.buylocalfood.com

- Organic Pages Online
  www.theorganicpages.com

ASK YOURSELF...

- How will eating organic foods contribute to my overall health?

- Where can I purchase organic foods nearby?

- Do I know which products are more important to buy organic?

- Can I spot the certified organic logos?

- Do I understand how the PLU system indicates how food is grown?

- Where can I buy local fresh produce and meats?

YOUR WELLNESS STRATEGIES

- Next time you pick up groceries, compare conventional to organic food prices.

- Look for the organic certification logos.

- Ask your grocer/butcher where they get their fruits, vegetables and meats.

- Buy local as much as you can – look on the Internet for a market near you or a delivery service.

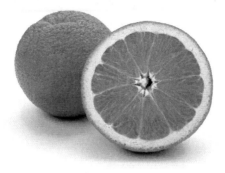

Chapter 11: Do We Need Multivitamins?
Are They All Created Equal?

– Dr. Nathalie

"Facts are stubborn things."

– Smollett

Our bodies are bombarded every day by biochemical stresses such as pesticides, herbicides, preservatives, genetically modified foods and fast foods that we eat on the run or at home because time is so precious for all of us. One way to make sure our bodies are getting the nutrients they need is to supplement our diet with high-quality vitamins and minerals.

Vitamins are organic compounds vital to our bodies' basic function. They play an important role as co-factors in numerous enzyme reactions in our body. Since our bodies can't manufacture vitamins, they need to be ingested through diet or by supplements. Vitamins help regulate our metabolism, help fight infection, repair and grow body tissues, give us energy and make us fertile. They even make us look good by making our hair shiny and thick, our nails strong, our teeth healthy and our skin youthful.

The following information is designed to give you some basic guidelines for buying and consuming multivitamins. It is not meant as a prescription for certain vitamins. Because we are all different and we all have different needs, your natural health care provider can best recommend vitamins and supplements that are specifically suited to you.

First, ask yourself these questions:

- Do I know why I should take vitamin supplements?
- Do I know which vitamins I should take?
- Do I know what brands have the highest nutritional quality?
- Is a multivitamin enough for me?

Here's another question for you: How much manganese did you take in yesterday? You probably don't know what that is or what it does for your body. Unfortunately, even if you think you eat fairly well, you don't necessarily know if you're covering all of your nutrient needs on a daily basis. In an ideal world, it would be best to get all the nutrients we need from high quality, wholesome food, but how realistic is that? With our busy lifestyles, we often don't take the time to plan and prepare well-balanced, nutritional meals. If you want to "cover your bases", taking a broad-spectrum nutritional supplement will ensure you get the right nutrients and it will help you protect yourself. Each vitamin and mineral plays an important role in maintaining your body's normal functions, repairing cellular and tissue damage and maintaining your optimal wellness.

Another reason why we don't get the needed nutrients from our everyday foods is that the earth's soils don't have the same nutritional values they once did; even as recently as 60 years ago. Nitrogen, phosphorus and potassium fertilizers have played a big role in depleting our soils of essential nutrients, and when nutrients aren't in our soil, they won't be found in our food.

The messages surrounding multivitamins have changed dramatically over the years. Twenty years ago experts were telling us *not* to take multivitamins if our diets were healthy as they were a waste of money. Research is now showing that more than 80 percent of the American population is not eating their daily recommended serving of fruits and vegetables.

Fat-soluble and Water-soluble Vitamins

Without getting into all the details of the vitamins' individual roles, know that there are 13 essential vitamins: thiamine (B1), riboflavin (B2), niacin/niacinamid (B3), pantothenic acid (B5), pyrodoxal/pyridoxamine/pyridoxine (B6), cobalamin (B12), biotin, folic acid, ascorbic acid (vitamin C), retinol/retinal/retinoic acid (vitamin A), calcitriol (active vitamin D form), tocopherols/tocotrienols (vitamin E family) and menaquinone (vitamin K active form).

Vitamins are categorized as either water soluble or fat soluble. Fat-soluble vitamins (A, D, E and K), are stored in the fat tissues in your body and your liver until your body needs them. They can be stored for a few days or sometimes even months. Water-soluble vitamins, like C and B, are easily excreted and are therefore hard to consume in toxic amounts. They must be replenished daily. Deficiencies can also occur if you have a pre-existing disease that prevents the food in your intestines from being absorbed properly. Alcoholism, multiple pregnancies and lactation can also deplete vitamins from your body. Many people suffer from micro-deficiencies, which may not show drastic symptoms. However, the deficiencies may eventually manifest as difficulty concentrating, lack of energy, headaches, etc. It's important not to ignore these symptoms. Even with vitamin supplementation, don't expect to see instant results. It could take time to get your body healthy again, depending on how deficient it has become. Unfortunately, some vitamin deficiencies can't always be reversed by reintroducing the vitamin to your diet.

Minerals also perform essential functions. They are divided in two groups: major mineral and trace minerals. Major minerals are: sodium, potassium, calcium, phosphorus, magnesium, chloride, and sulfur. These minerals are generally required in amounts greater then 100mg per day. Trace minerals are: iron, zinc, manganese, fluoride, iodine, selenium, copper, molybdenum and chromium. These minerals are needed in only microgram amounts.

Not all Vitamins Are Created Equal

Not all vitamins are created equal, quality is the key! In the book, The Comparative Guide to Nutritional Supplements, by Dr. Lyle MacWilliam, over 1,500 supplements available in Canada and the United States were evaluated. Each supplement was given a *Health Support Profile* based on 18 criteria – completeness, potency, mineral forms, bioactivity of vitamin E, gammatocopherol, antioxidant support, bone health, heart health, liver health, metabolic health, ocular health, methylation support, lipotrophic factors, inflammation control, glycation control, bioflavonoid profile, phenolic compound profile and potential toxicities. Each product was then given a score based on a star system (zero stars to five stars) with five stars being the best. When I show the book to my patients they are shocked to see that the multivitamin they have been taking for years scored .5 stars out of five! It is important to note that the guide is a non-sponsored publication.

According to <u>The Comparative Guide to Nutritional Supplements</u>, most vitamins found in drug stores – even recognized brands – have a very low absorption rate. In contrast, high quality vitamins, often available through a natural health provider, can provide you with an absorption rate of close to 100 percent. So the question is: would you rather pay $10 for vitamins that only let you retain three to 10 percent of the nutritional value, or spend a little more money for vitamins that let you retain 100 percent of the nutritional value? It's a no-brainer to me!

Since nutrients do not work in isolation but rather work with each other, a good supplement will ensure proper ratios to help you absorb the most nutrients. A good vitamin supplement manufacturer will also ensure that the binders and expedients used are not harmful to your health. There are a lot of 'one-a-day' multivitamins on drugstore shelves. In order to compress all the needed vitamins into one tablet, it requires a lot of binders, which are hard to digest or absorb and are sometimes even toxic. That is why with good quality vitamins, you'll often have to take more than one a day. But remember, convenience shouldn't win over quality.

Take note as well that regulations for vitamins made in Canada are more stringent than those in the U.S. (not to say that the U.S. doesn't have great vitamins). Canadian regulations fall under pharmaceutical guidelines and therefore have a higher standard than those in the U.S., which fall under more lenient food regulation guidelines. Food-grade supplements may contain a wide array of unhealthy binders and fillers, including petroleum products, coal tar derivatives, shampoos, sands – the list goes on.

In addition, because they are considered foods and not drugs, the American Food and Drug Administration (FDA), does not monitor the content of the supplements or the source of the nutrition ingredient. In Canada, supplements need to be more than 99 percent pure to be on the Canadian market, so the purity and potency is much higher. The con to this, however, is that, in Canada, due to the strict regulations, it can take seemingly forever to get a great supplement approved for sale. Safety and performance should always be the bottom line, so do your due diligence and get the proper information on the vitamins you are taking!

According to the Comparative Guide, the Top-ranked Vitamins Are:

- Creating Wellness™
- Douglas Laboratories

- Truestar Health
- USANA Health Science

It's Important to Know…

- Your multivitamins should be manufactured at an International Organization for Standardization (ISO) or National Sanitation Foundation (NSF) certified facility to confirm that the product is made using the highest standards available;

- Look for a multivitamin certified GMP (Good Manufacturing Practice) to ensure that what is said to be on the label is in the bottle—nothing more, nothing less.

- Some binder ingredients in a vitamin could make the vitamins themselves harder to absorb and digest;

- Vitamins and minerals should be taken with food as they are harder to digest on an empty stomach and might make you nauseous.

Taking a poor supplement can be worse than taking no supplement at all. Not only do you get a sense of false security about getting adequate nutrition but, depending on the supplement's fillers, you can also be ingesting toxic substances.

I believe the regulations surrounding vitamins and supplements need to be reviewed. We need to create better evaluation systems and communications around this important topic as it has the potential to extend our lifespan and could save our health care system millions of dollars. One of the challenges with this issue is that many consumers have been brainwashed into thinking "natural" means "healthy." Sure, some products are "natural" but what about the quality and the safety of the ingredients? We have to be very aware and careful about what we put into our bodies, even if it's called "natural," and whether or not it's sold off the shelf or bought online! We have to do our due diligence not only for our multivitamins but also for all other supplements.

Note on whole food vitamins – whole food vitamins are rapidly gaining in popularity. Whole food vitamins are—as the name implies—vitamins made from whole foods. New natural technologies are making supplements more effective by allowing better absorption of the nutrients by the body. Keep in mind that regular vitamins are tested according to pharmaceutical grade testing standards. Whole food vitamins are tested by professional grade nutritional standards.

ASK YOURSELF...

- How do I know if I am getting the right amount of vitamins and minerals from my food?

- Should I be taking a multivitamin to complement my diet?

- Do I know the quality of my current multivitamin?

- Where can I find a high quality vitamin?

YOUR WELLNESS STRATEGIES

- Consult a natural health care provider to determine your nutritional needs.

- Research the quality of the supplements you are currently taking by looking them up in the book, <u>The Comparative Guide to Nutritional Supplements</u>.

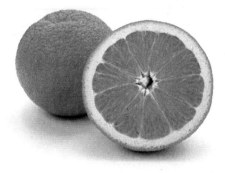

Chapter 12: The Power Of Omega-3

– Dr. Nathalie

"A discovery is said to be an accident meeting a prepared mind."
– Albert Szent-Gyorgyo

Do you remember when you were young and your parents forced you to take fish oil by the teaspoon, saying that it was good for you? Guess what? They were right!

Omega-3 and Omega-6 are called essential fatty acids (EFAs) and are poly-unsaturated fats. Since your body cannot manufacture EFAs, they need to be obtained from the food you eat or the supplements you take. Linoleic Acid (LA) is a primary member of the Omega-6 fatty acids and can be found in leafy vegetables, seeds, nuts, grains, and vegetable oils like corn oil, soybean oil, sunflower oil. Vegetarian diets tend to be very high in Omega-6.

Omega-3 fatty acids have three main types. The first two, EPA (eicosapentaenoic acid) and DHA (docosahexanoic acid), are both found in cold water fish. Fresh seaweed is the only plant food that contains a significant amount of EPA and DHA. The third type of Omega-3, called ALA (alpha-linolenic acid), is found in oils (like flaxseed), although small amounts can also be found in some nuts and seeds. In order for your body to benefit from DHA and EPA, your body must be able to convert the ALA to DHA and EPA. Your body may not always be able to make that conversion if your organs are not working as efficiently as they should, therefore, the only way to truly ensure your body gets the powerhouse benefits of DHA and EPA is to take it directly in the form of fish oil.

Most North Americans currently consume between 20 and 50 times more Omega-6 than Omega-3, although for optimal health, the ratio should be about 3:1. As you can see from this ratio, most people don't need to supplement with Omega-6; since they already get enough from their diet. Science is now pointing to the fact that a major cause of the current high incidence of heart disease, hypertension, diabetes, obesity and some forms of cancer is the imbalance between Omega-6 and Omega-3.

Many ailments or diseases can be traced back to a deficiency in Omega-3 fatty acids, they have been shown to support a healthy cholesterol level along with musculoskeletal, cardiovascular, endocrine and immune system functions. Research shows that imbalances between Omega-6 and Omega-3 fatty acids can increase inflammation, coagulation and the growth of adipose and cancer cells.

Fish oil has also been shown to play a crucial role in weight loss. Fish oils turn on your lipolytic (fat burning) genes, turns off the lipogenic (fat storage) genes and increases the use of fat stores from your adiposities (fat cells).

Other Benefits of Fish Oil Include:

- Promotion of good heart health
- Decrease in triglycerides and high blood pressure
- Enhancement of circulation
- Decrease in depression
- Reduction of symptoms of Attention Deficit Hyperactive Disorder
- Better memory, learning and help with Alzheimer's Disease
- Reduction of allergies
- Clearer skin
- Reduction of inflammation from arthritis
- Regulation of insulin
- Improvement of immune system health
- Better women's reproductive health

- Enhancement of vision

- Reduction of inflammatory bowel disease

As mentioned earlier, the most efficient way to ensure that you get DHA and EPA is to take it directly in the form of fish oil. While I usually espouse the value of getting your nutrients directly from the source, cold water fish, unfortunately, often contains metals that are harmful to humans, such as mercury. Therefore getting your Omega-3 from fish oil supplements might be a healthier option, especially if you don't know the origin of the fish you're buying.

Adding Omega-3 to your diet is important. If you opt for a fish oil supplement be very careful of the source. Look for fish oil that:

- Is pharmaceutical-grade

- Is third party certified for purity and quality

- Has an antioxidant blend for freshness and stability

- Is free from pesticides and heavy metals such as mercury, PCBs and dioxins

- Is custom-made in small batch production

The antioxidant in fish oil is important because it is perishable. The antioxidants are needed so that the fish oil does not oxidize in your body, causing free radicals that are hazardous to your health. High-quality fish oil supplements are stabilized with adequate amounts of antioxidants. To help protect the fat in the oil from oxidation, 400 units of vitamin E is commonly used.

Once you've decided to take these supplements, your next question is likely how much should you take? There are no set amounts for this supplement. Different people will require different amounts, depending on diet and physical condition. Be aware, however, that studies show no additional health benefits *above* five grams/day of EPA and DHA combined. Consult your natural health care provider to determine your specific needs.

Also, when choosing your fish oil supplement, know that cod liver oil and fish oil are not the same. Cod liver oil is extracted from the liver of cod fish, and contains lower levels of EPA and DHA. Cod liver oil is also very high in vitamins D and A, so if you are exposed to a lot of sun you could overdose on vitamin D. If you decide to eat more fish to obtain your Omega-3, try to buy natural fish rather than farmed fish. Farmed fish are grown in captivity and can contain the same growth hormones as farmed chicken and beef, raised solely for the purpose of profit. Choosing natural fish is better for you and also for the environment. If you are concerned about the mercury levels in fish, I recommend you visit www.gotmercury.com. As a basic rule, the smaller the fish the better it is. Bigger fish have more time to accumulate a higher level of toxicity from the polluted ocean floor.

The research showing the health benefits of Omega-3 fatty acids is compelling. It is also important to note that Omega-6 has pro-inflammatory properties and should be limited, as opposed to Omega-3 which has anti-inflammatory properties. This is one of the many reasons to supplement with Omega-3; a lot of current health concerns are caused by inflammatory conditions such as heart disease and arthritis, to name a few.

You don't necessarily have to take your supplement in liquid form (I know I can't). Several quality companies offer great encapsulated fish oils, some of which are lemon coated so you won't even taste the fish when you swallow nor when you digest. It is always better to take supplements with food for easier digestion. If for some reason, you choose not to take fish oil supplementation because you do not want to consume fish, or are concerned about contaminants or toxicity, you can select a vegetable alternative. You may also have environmental concerns about over-fishing and sustainability. As discussed earlier, people are consuming more Omega-6 than Omega-3. This creates a disproportioned ratio, which may lead to disease. So be certain that your vegetable sources are high in Omega-3.

ASK YOURSELF...

- Am I taking fish oil daily to enhance my health and wellness?

- If I do take a fish oil supplement, am I using a quality product?

- Does the product I'm taking contain antioxidants to prevent oxidation in my body?

YOUR WELLNESS STRATEGIES

- Decide this week to begin a fish oil regime.

- Do your due diligence and find a high quality Omega-3 supplement.

- Find a naturopathic doctor, chiropractor, nutritionist or another natural health care provider who can recommend a quality product.

- Once opened, keep your bottle refrigerated for quality and freshness. Be aware of the expiry date.

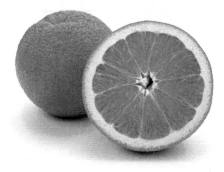

Chapter 13: Looking At Stress Creatively

– Andrée

"You don't drown by falling in the water; you drown by staying there."
– Edwin Louis-Cole

Have you ever noticed how the very things in life we think are demons can turn out to be gifts? Take stress, for example. Everyone experiences stress from time to time, some more than others. There are two ways to look at stress – as something that is unavoidable in our hectic lives, or something we can embrace and learn from, maybe even master. Our responses to positive and negative stressors determine a huge part of our wellness, but what exactly is stress, and where does it come from?

It might help to understand the different kinds of stress and what their origins are:

- Eustress – a type of stress that is fun, exciting, and keeps you alert e.g. skiing down a slope, bungee jumping, skydiving or some other kind of extreme sport; it is self-inflicted;

- Acute stress – a very short-term type of stress that you encounter sometime during the day that can be either positive or negative – from racing to meet a deadline to dealing with road rage;

- Episodic acute stress – a kind of stress that runs rampant and becomes a way of life, creating a cycle of relative chaos – this is the type of stress that turns someone into a "drama queen" or "absent-minded professor";

- Chronic stress – a stress that seems never-ending and inescapable like the stress of financial troubles, an unfulfilling marriage or an extremely taxing job. This type of stress can eventually lead to burnout or worse, chronic illness or disease.

I bet that while you were reading these definitions, something inside of you started to stir. Maybe a lot or maybe just a flicker. The point is that one or more of these definitions probably resonated on some level with you, as they do with all of us. The question is; what type(s) of stress do you have in your life and what is it doing to your emotional, physical and spiritual state of well-being? Identifying the type of stresses you are experiencing in your life and the length of time that you experience them, will determine your overall state of health and well-being.

"Stress becomes a problem when there's too much, when it lasts too long or when it comes too often."

– David Posen, MD

The symptoms you experience when you feel stressed can be:

- Mental – memory loss, lack of focus, lack of concentration and confusion;

- Emotional – crying, moodiness, inappropriate laughter, uncontrollable anger, despondency and even depression;

- Physical – sleeplessness, sleeping too much, lack of appetite or increased appetite, physical tension, various aches and pains such as recurring headaches and poor digestion;

- Behavioral – lack of interest in your usual activities, irrational behavior such as making rash decisions or the inability to make a decision at all.

Anything sound familiar here? Everyone experiences stress at different levels and with varying symptoms. So how do you know when the stress in your life is getting out of control and what you can do about it when it does?

STRESS:
Solving
Tension
Relevant to
Events,
Situations and
Self!

Welcome to your new way of dealing with stress. Write this down and post it everywhere you can think of – your fridge, your desk, your car. I want you to change your definition of stress. What a powerful thing to realize that you can master the stress in your life just by how you perceive it. And by changing the way you perceive it, you give it an appropriate amount of power instead of letting it rule you! Breaking down this new way of thinking even further, start by identifying where your stress originates.

Once you've pinpointed what's been stressing you, realize that it's your *perception* of events and situations that drive your stress barometer reading up or down. The way we react to stressful situations and events usually comes from a learned behavior or some kind of internal dialogue as we've discussed in previous chapters – perhaps even from our parents. Take thunderstorms, for example, the fear and stress of thunderstorms can actually be passed on from generation to generation, if you let it. Or, we can recognize where that fear might be coming from, own that feeling and choose not to give that fear so much power. Whatever the situation, remember: it's not *what* happens to you, it's *how* you deal with it that makes your stress level go up or down.

If you have a stressful situation in your life that keeps coming up, over and over again, take a moment to center yourself and visualize the way you'd like to handle that situation the next time it comes around. Remember, you are in the driver's seat here. The worst thing you can do with stress is deny or ignore it. Dealing with stress takes creativity; the more creative you are in dealing with stress when it comes your way, the more control you'll have and the better you'll feel. Own your circumstances.

Here are some other tricks to de-stress creatively and take ownership of a stressful situation:

Laughter

Laughing can actually make you live longer. Doctors have known for years that humor can help cure disease, especially in very sick children, which is why there are so many clowns and other performers at hospitals for sick children.

There are many benefits to laughter, including reducing stress, provoking relaxation, lowering blood pressure and improving brain function. This last benefit is particularly important in times of stress, because we have to be able to choose how we are going to respond to stress in the moment. So, anything we can do to increase our chances of doing that effectively can only be good. Force a hearty laugh if you have to and after a while your body will take over naturally (see chapter #27 – "Laughter Is The Sunshine Of Your Life").

Physical Activity

Physical activity is a great way to reduce stress. Any activity that you enjoy, that brings you a sense of well-being or simply gives you time for yourself, will be beneficial. Try yoga, go for a walk, go for a run and dance, dance, dance to your favorite tunes. Find an activity or hobby you are passionate about, that involves some kind of movement, and go for it.

Talk

We all need someone to talk to. Do you have a special friend or confidante, someone who can be objective, who can listen when you just need to share? You might also want to consider hiring a life coach to help you sift through some of your negative patterns. They can suggest what shifts you need to make so that your life is less stressful. Sometimes, the help of a good therapist might be required as well. Don't be afraid to seek help.

Notice your self-talk – your inner conversations as we mentioned above. What are you saying to yourself when you first get up in the morning? Do you embrace the day with conviction and confidence or do you feel defeated before you have even started? First of all, don't beat yourself up about it. That's why you're reading this book, to learn how to break those negative patterns and grow. If you're thinking negatively upon waking, take a moment to recognize that, own it, and think about ways to let go of that stress-inducing behavior. Ask yourself whether or not you talk to yourself the way you would like others to speak to you – with kindness, compassion, love and respect.

Create Anchors

Create memories that will serve as anchors to support you in stressful times. Refer to those good memories when you need them. Whether a favorite vacation spot or the image of a precious pet or even a soothing song – use those anchors to ground you and get you through the stress.

Be in the Moment

Carpe Diem, Seize the Day! In fact, seize each moment! If you're present in all that you do, all that you see, all that you hear, and you see the beauty in life, you won't have as much time to worry and be stressed. Take time to enjoy the food you eat and to hear the laughter around you. The splendor of it will allow you to let stress simply slide off your shoulders. Remember, it's all about perception.

Balance

Add balance to your life. When was the last time you took time for you? Read a few pages of a novel, take a hot bubble bath, give yourself an organic facial or look at old photographs. Invest in time for you. It will pay off.

Be Willing Not to Know

Sometimes, particularly as parents, we feel we have to know the answers to everything. No one knows everything about everything. Give yourself permission to be human, to not have the answer or solution to every problem or dilemma and be comfortable with that. If you think about it, you may even be empowering someone else in your life to grow if you challenge them to explore their own solutions; and what a beautiful gift that would be for both of you.

If you need an answer to an internal question, it will come eventually. Don't stress out about it or force yourself to come up with an answer upon request.

ASK YOURSELF...

- What areas of my life are stressing me out?

- How stressful is my financial situation?

- How much stress are my primary relationships causing me?

- Is my health and wellness a cause of stress for me?

- Am I happy in my job, my career?

- Am I overdoing it at work or at home?

- Is there too much on my schedule or too little?

- Do I feel I'm on my way to a burnout?

YOUR WELLNESS STRATEGIES

- Do one thing this week to take better care of yourself.

- Take one action this week to better manage your stress.

- Take one action this week to make a positive difference in your life.

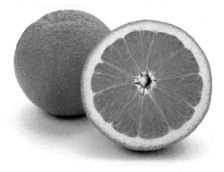

Chapter 14: Deodorant – Sometimes The Facts Stink

– Dr. Nathalie

"Knowledge is power."

– Sir Francis Bacon

We all sweat, so it's not surprising that 90 percent of us regularly use antiperspirants and deodorants. In fact, sales of these products are only exceeded by one other bathroom staple – toothpaste.

You likely use deodorant to mask underarm odor or use antiperspirants to reduce sweating. Unfortunately, health concerns over both are growing. If you have to use one, go with a deodorant. Antiperspirants clog and close your pores, inhibiting you from sweating; this is not a normal or healthy thing.

While deodorant is a better choice than antiperspirant, there is some evidence that the chemicals used in both products may be contributing to a higher incidence of breast cancer. Studies show a disproportionately large number of breast cancer cases in the upper outer quadrant of the breast; precisely where deodorant and antiperspirant are usually applied. Studies are showing that breast cancer incidences rose at a similar rate as deodorant/antiperspirant sales. It is, however, important to note that there is no *conclusive* evidence to prove there is a relationship between breast cancer and deodorants...

What Should You Watch For When Buying Deodorant?

It is suggested not to put anything on your skin that you wouldn't eat! The dreadful truth is that more than a third of our personal care products contain ingredients that have been linked in some way to cancer and according to the Environmental Working Group, only 11 percent of the 10,500 ingredients used have ever been tested for safety. This is because neither Canada nor the U.S. has a mandate to safeguard the cosmetics industry. With nearly 4,000,000 synthetic chemicals out there, it seems too daunting a task. Have a look at chapter #34 "Cosmetics – Painting A Different Picture", for a more detailed list of chemicals you should avoid. Here are the most common chemicals used in deodorants that you should avoid buying:

Aluminum – One main concern with deodorants is related to their high levels of aluminum salts. Aluminum chloride, aluminum carbohydrate and aluminum zirconium chlorhydrate glycine complexes can make up 25 percent of the weight of the deodorant/antiperspirant, which is not healthy – especially in Western cultures where most women shave their underarms, resulting in more skin absorption of the harmful substances. Aluminum has also been linked to Alzheimer's disease.

Parabens – These are another concern related to deodorants. Parabens may be listed on labels as: methyl parabens, ethyl parabens, propyl parabens, butyl parabens, isobutyl parabens or E216. These parabens have shown particularly troubling links to cancer, present and intact in breast tumors. Studies have also shown that parabens affect the body much like estrogens do – diminishing muscle mass, allowing for extra storage of fat and prompting male gynecomastia (breast growth).

Propylene Glycol – found in thousands of cosmetic products – to help moisturize. It is also an ingredient used in anti-freeze and brake fluid, so it's no surprise that it could cause liver abnormalities and kidney damage.

Fragrance – found in many deodorants. While it may seem harmless, it should be avoided as it can cause allergies and lung problems. Unfortunately, the priority of most companies that sell beauty products is their financial bottom line, not your long-term health. Ultimately, we can't ignore the fact that all the chemicals we use on our body may increase our risk of developing cancer. Knowledge is power, but you have to act on that knowledge.

To protect yourself, here are a few things you can do:

- Don't apply deodorant right after shaving underarms

- Avoid application if there are open cuts

- Read labels and look for a more natural deodorant

- Keep your body alkaline. Oral chlorophyll tablets can help reduce body odor and can eliminate the need for deodorants

Healthier Alternatives

Baking soda powder – Take a pinch of baking soda powder in one hand. Drop several drops of water on it, blend and then rub under arms. You'll be amazed how effective it is!

Natural Mineral salts – a natural mineral salt deodorant stick will improve your skin's Ph level while protecting against odor-causing bacteria.

Natural deodorant – natural health food stores will carry deodorants that don't have harmful chemicals.

Au Natural – consider not using any deodorant! If you feed your body the right food and keep your body alkaline, you may not actually need it. Give it a try. People around you will hopefully let you know!

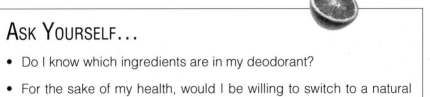

Ask Yourself...

- Do I know which ingredients are in my deodorant?

- For the sake of my health, would I be willing to switch to a natural product?

- Would I be willing to re-apply the natural deodorant during the day rather than using harmful chemicals once per day?

YOUR WELLNESS STRATEGIES

- Check your deodorant label to see if they contain aluminum, parabens or propylene glycol.

- Schedule a trip to a health food store and look into a healthier personal care product.

- Share your knowledge with your friends and pass on good health!

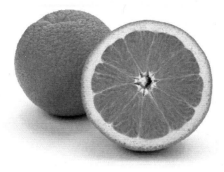

Chapter 15: Breathe Clean

– Dr. Nathalie

"We are so busy doing the urgent that we don't have time to do the important."

– Confusius

"The air within homes and other buildings can be more seriously polluted than the outdoor air in even the largest and most industrialized cities."

– U.S. Environmental Protection Agency

You can't control the pollution when you step outside, but you can definitely have some control over the quality of the air you breathe inside your home and office.

North Americans spend an average of 90 percent of their time inside, but their indoor environments may be full of toxic substances in the air they breathe. Research shows that exposure to indoor contaminants can be 2 to 100 times higher than the contaminants outside. You might be thinking that your house is clean and not polluted, but in all likelihood it is. This, of course, is hazardous to your health.

Chemicals, Natural Allergens and Pollutants Hiding in Your Home

- Construction materials like lead, formaldehyde and paint;

- Solvents, insecticides, herbicides and disinfectants from household products you use regularly;

- Dust, dander and chemicals on carpets, clothes and bedding;

- Food waste, cooking odors and vapors in the kitchen;

- Pollen, mould, hair and skin in air vents;

- Sewer gas and mildew in the bathroom.

All these contaminants can have an effect on your health if present in high enough quantities and, if you are exposed to them day in and day out.

Major Health Problems Related to Indoor Air Pollution

- Asthma;

- Sick Building Syndrome (SBS) – This may take time to notice because the symptoms resolve themselves once you leave the area and come back upon return. SBS can involve health problems with multiple systems of the body including headaches, nausea, eye, throat and skin irritation;

- Multiple Chemical Sensitivity – This is when your body negatively responds to low-levels of chemicals that are commonly found in indoor environments. Symptoms are similar to SBS and commonly fade when you leave the environment that's making you ill, although for some people, symptoms persist outside the environment;

- Hypersensitivity Pneumonitis – This is caused by bacteria, fungi and moulds that are contaminating home humidifiers, heating, ventilation and air conditioning systems. The symptoms are flu-like and include chills, fever, fatigue, cough, chest tightness and shortness of breath. This is usually reversible when regular exposure to the harmful environment is halted.

Possible Symptoms of SBS, MCS and general indoor air pollution:

- Headache

- Eye and throat irritation

- Chest tightness

- Shortness of breath

- Fatigue

- Nausea

- Skin irritation

Air Cleaners

Air cleaning devices are either central filtration systems, often called in-duct systems, placed into the heating, ventilation, and air conditioning system of a home, or portable units with an attached fan. Portable units help clean the air in a single room while central air units can improve the air throughout a home.

Below is a list of a variety of air cleaners and their attributes:

- **Mechanical Filters** – These filters draw air through a flat, pleated or high efficiency particulate to trap particles.

- **Hepa Filters** – The most efficient mechanical filters for removing small particles that can be breathed deep into the lungs. The highest efficiency mechanical filters available today are up to 99.97 percent effective and can remove particles just 0.3 microns in size. One micron = 1 millionth of a meter.

- **Electronic Air Cleaners** – There are three general types of electric air cleaning technologies:

  1. Ozone generator technology:

     Watch out for air cleaners that clean by producing ozone. Ozone in the upper atmosphere protects you from the sun's ultraviolet rays, but ground-level ozone is an irritant that can aggravate asthma and hinder lung function. Ozone, at this level, is a harmful air pollutant and can affect the respiratory system of children, the elderly, asthmatics and those with respiratory problems the most. Long-term effects of ozone can also reduce the average person's breathing ability. Studies have shown that 50 ppb should be your maximum exposure to ozone, but it's better to avoid it altogether. Public health authorities have started to forbid the use of machines that produce ozone.

  2. Electrostatic precipitator technology:

     Electrostatic precipitator technology uses a small electrical charge to collect particles from air pulled through the device (charged plate electrical system). A major drawback of this technology is that because there is no fan, air doesn't circulate as much, making it less than efficient. This process produces some ozone as a by-product of the ion-generating technology they use.

3.   Ionizers or negative ion generator technology:

First of all, let's explain what negative ions are because even the word "negative" makes you think they are not healthy and that is simply not the case. Negative ions are produced by oxygen atoms and help provide a feeling of fresh air. High amounts of these ions are found in natural environments like forests and waterfalls. Negative ions also create a soothing, relaxing atmosphere as if you were surrounded by nature. Household air conditioners reduce the number of negative ions present in an indoor environment so an ion generator can help correct this imbalance. So having negative ions in our air is good! Now let's talk about the technology. Ionizers work by causing particles to stick to materials near the ionizer (carpet and wall), taking them out of the air we breathe. Not only does this process produce ozone as a by-product, it does not necessarily clean the air of the particles created, which could easily become loose again and re-circulate.

A better and safer type of negative ion technology is called a clean ion generator. This adds negative ions after mechanical filtering, not as part of the filtering process, which would use the negative ions to attract particles. The negative ions are added after to give the health benefits of recreating a healthier air and environment, all without the unwanted effect of ozone production.

Photo Catalytic Oxidation Technology

Another newer type of electronic air cleaner technology is called photo catalytic oxidation (PCO) with ultraviolet light. PCO technology uses ultraviolet light to help clean the air. If you decide to choose PCO technology, make sure that the units do not create ozone in the process.

Some hybrid air cleaners are available which combine the different technologies, but again be aware that electronic air cleaning produces ozone and there is no real safe amount of ozone!

Take notes on...

- Portable Air Cleaners – These cleaners can replace the air in a room two to three times every hour. The effectiveness of portable air cleaners is often rated in terms of pollutant removal efficiency or 'Clean Air Delivery Rate' (CADR). CADR ratings are given separately for the removal of dust, pollen and environmental tobacco smoke. Any portable air cleaner with a CADR score above 350 is excellent and below 100 is poor.

- Central System Air Cleaners – These systems change the air in a room about every two hours. To ensure you get the most air-flow possible, have your system's ductwork pressure-tested for leakage and then sealed and insulated. This should be done by an experienced heating and ventilating contractor.

Tips to Breathing Better Indoor Air

- Use a high-efficiency filter in your central heating/cooling system with at least a 60 percent efficiency grade. This will help remove harmful airborne particles;

- Minimize the humidity in your home by letting more outdoor air in and ensuring sufficient ventilation. By doing this, you'll prevent moisture from building up on walls and windows, reducing the possible growth of bacteria. You may need to buy a ceiling fan to optimize air-flow in highly humid areas;

- Measure the humidity in your home by using a hygrometer – you can get an inexpensive one at a hardware store. The relative humidity in your home should be below 50 percent in the summer and below 30 percent in the winter. If your home doesn't achieve this on its own you should invest in a dehumidifier;

- Repair leaky roofs, walls and foundations;

- Clean frequently and thoroughly to prevent dust and mould build up;

- Regularly clean and disinfect filters of furnaces, humidifiers, de-humidifiers and air conditioners;

- Keep aerosol product use to a minimum;

- Restrict smoking to outdoor areas or, better yet, just quit!

- Use exhaust fans that vent to the outdoors when cooking;

- When purchasing building materials and furniture, choose products that do not emit formaldehyde – ask a sales person/manufacturer when in doubt;

- Carefully follow safety instructions on consumer products such as cleaning agents, paints and glues;

- Consider using chemical-free cleaning products. There are several on the market now (good for you and the environment!);

- Consider using micro-fiber cleaning cloths with embedded silver. This technology allows you to clean your house with no cleaning agents;

- Limit the use of candles and incense indoors as they can elevate indoor particle levels;

- Use plenty of ventilation.

Do your due diligence when investing in an air purifying system; they are often a significant investment and you want the highest quality for the best price. There is one product I personally use and recommend for purifying the air in your home – the Nikken Air Wellness Power5 Pro. It has a 5-stage mechanical filtration system, is ozone-free, Energy Star certified and produces negative ions *after* the filtering process as opposed to during. For more information, visit www.nikken.com.

ASK YOURSELF...

- Do I know what type of air filter I'm using in my home?

- Do I limit indoor pollutants by choosing healthy products for my home?

- Do I have health symptoms mentioned in this chapter and could they be due to my home air environment?

Your Wellness Strategies

- Check your furnace's filter; does it need to be changed? Is it high-efficiency?

- From now on, try to buy mostly chemical free products.

- Consider replacing your carpets with floating or hardwood flooring. Be aware of the chemicals used to stain your floors.

- Research different portable air systems to improve the quality of the air you breathe indoors or at least in the rooms where you spend most of your time!

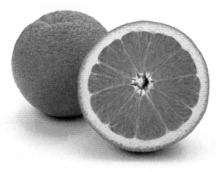

Chapter 16: Just Breathe

– Andrée

"It is my experience that natural breathing is in itself a powerful form of self-healing."
– Dennis Lewis, "The Tao of Natural Breathing"

Why is breathing so important? Simply put, you need to breathe to stay alive. All living things need to breathe to stay alive – plants, animals and humans.

Try this: take a few deep breaths (without raising your shoulders) and feel your ribcage expand and contract. This simple action opens up your lungs so that air is taken into them and oxygen is pumped to your blood. That oxygen is then carried throughout your body, to your heart, brain, digestive system and so on. This keeps you alive and well.

Effects of Not Breathing Right

When your body doesn't get enough oxygen you feel sluggish, tired and groggy. If your breathing is too shallow and too quick, you will find yourself hyperventilating due to anxiety and actually end up with an excess of oxygen and not enough carbon dioxide in your blood which is equally detrimental to your health. This imbalance in blood gases can do everything from making your fingertips tingle to causing dizziness and even faintness.

Breathing is vital and breathing properly is a key to good health. Learning how to breathe more naturally, the way your body was designed to breathe, can have a powerful influence on your overall health and metabolism. Breathing is a fundamental force that has subtle inter-relationships with many different parts of you – your body, mind, emotions and spirit.

Watch how a baby breathes for the perfect example of proper breathing. Healthy babies breathe so naturally, without effort, without thought. The chest and abdomen rise and fall as the baby breathes in and then out, taking in oxygen and releasing carbon dioxide. Many people need to re-learn how to breathe naturally. Sedentary work environments, inactive lifestyle and the ever-increasing stress of busy lives have conditioned so many people to breathe in a shallow, constricted way, simply in the upper chest. Poor breathing like this can decrease your vitality and increase mental and emotional stress. It's important to ensure that you re-learn how to breathe properly, using the full range of movement in your lungs, diaphragm, belly and back to inhale and exhale freely and fully. Through natural, authentic breathing, you will reduce stress, improve your health and increase your energy.

Natural and Nose Breathing

Natural breathing is also known as "whole-body breathing", because it involves so many parts of you. With natural breathing, the depth and speed of inhalation and exhalation are directly proportionate to the demands being placed on the body. This type of breathing is done through the nose, so the hairs in your nose filter out dust and dirt particles that your mouth and throat cannot. Nose breathing also warms and moisturizes the air. This is breathing at its best! Yoga has traditionally taught that breathing through the nose maintains the correct balance of oxygen and carbon dioxide in the blood and has a relaxing effect – when you feel more relaxed you can deal with stress more effectively.

Mouth Breathing

Mouth breathing expels carbon dioxide much too quickly therefore restricting the oxygen in the blood and consequently to the brain. As a result, you might feel tense, irritable and anxious, which is not conducive to your health.

Be Aware!

Start noticing how you are breathing. Put your hand on your stomach, does it expand and contract as you breathe? Or does just your chest rise and fall with each breath? To breathe more consciously and naturally, you might need to consider losing any excess weight you have. If you need to, start out slowly; try a brisk walk for at least 30 minutes a day during your lunch hour and then progress to a swimming or yoga class a couple of times a week. Exercise will help develop your natural breathing and make your body and mind healthier.*

Ask Yourself...

- Am I breathing deeply or shallowly?

- Do I often find myself breathing through my mouth?

- What one action can I take this week to teach myself to breathe better?

Your Wellness Strategies

- This week take five minutes every day to sit quietly and notice your breathing.

- Contemplate joining a yoga class to become more aware of your breathing.

- Go for a brisk walk, and notice how your breathing changes.

- If you feel stressed or anxious at any time this week, take a few moments to breathe in slowly and deeply through your nose and release the breath once again slowly through your nose. Do this four or five times and notice how you feel afterwards.

Note: Before you attempt any exercise program, please check with your doctor.

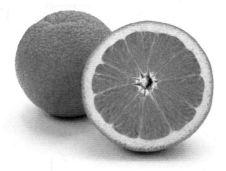

Chapter 17: Adjusting Your Inner PH For Optimal Health

– Dr. Nathalie

"One should eat to live, and not live to eat."
– Molière

I heard this story a few years ago and I really thought it was the perfect analogy for why we need to keep our bodies as healthy and balanced as possible. Imagine you have a big pile of garbage in your house. If you leave that pile of garbage long enough it will start to rot and it will attract vermin such as rats. So what could you do? You could call in the exterminator and he gets rid of the rats. So far so good, except if you don't clear away the garbage, the rats will come back and you'll be back to square one, right? Your problem was never the rats but the garbage that attracted them in the first place. The same is true for your body. If you don't give your body a clean, healthy environment in which to flourish, you are creating a kind of garbage dump which may very well attract disease if kept in that state long enough. You can try to get rid of disease in all sorts of ways but if you don't change the environment (your body), it will come back.

The book by Dr. Robert O. Young called, The pH Miracle, has provided solutions for many people with deteriorating health problems. The premise of the book is that an acidic pH level in the body can cause or continue to feed disease; but learning how to create a harmonious, balanced pH level in the body can do just the opposite.

"There is only one disease – the over-acidity of the fluids and tissues of the body which leads to an overgrowth of microorganisms whose toxic wastes produce the symptoms we call disease."

– Dr. Robert O. Young PH.D.

PH Levels

Most people are familiar with acid rain and the damage it does to our environment. Acid has a similar effect on the internal human environment. Therefore we need to become internal environmentalists and safeguard our internal health.

PH stands for "potential of hydrogen" and is the measure of how acidic or alkaline a substance is – pH levels range from 0 – 14, with 7 being neutral.

The normal pH of the body:

- Gastric acid = 1.0-2.0
- Normal urine = 6.0 to 6.5 in the morning
      6.5 to 7.0 in the evening
- Saliva = 6.5 to 7.5
- Blood = 7.4

When our pH level decreases, it signifies that our body is more acidic, and when it rises, our body is more alkaline. Litmus paper is a simple tool to measure and monitor your pH levels and is available at natural health food stores to test saliva pH and urine pH. Urine testing may be more reliable as saliva values are more difficult to interpret since they are impacted by digestive impairment and are influenced greatly by our blood. Please note that some authors do not agree with these methods of measurement as they might be too arbitrary. They suggest looking at the alkalinity or acidity of the food ingested to help you determine your alkaline-acid levels.

Several variables have to be taken into consideration when doing these kinds of tests – all ingested food and all situations (physical, emotional or mental) can play a role in acidity or alkalinity levels.

Acidity

In general, people are more likely to have an acidity imbalance rather than an alkaline imbalance. The Western diet can be very acidic with a lot of meat, sugar and processed foods. Tobacco, alcohol, coffee and low physical activity are also contributors to an acidic environment – and while we could counter this to some degree by eating more alkaline-producing foods like vegetables, these things are often times not as abundant as they should be on our grocery list.

Acid-forming reaction refers to any changes in the body that produce a decreased ability to energize the system and leave an acid residue in the urine. Acid-forming minerals found in food are: phosphorus, sulphur, chlorine, iodine, bromine, fluorine, copper and silicon.

When you have a highly acidic diet, it puts pressure on your body's regulating systems to work at achieving a neutral pH – this depletes your blood of the alkaline forming minerals like sodium, potassium, calcium and magnesium to act as buffers, and can lead to chronic and degenerative illnesses. In addition, disease – including cancer – thrives in acidic environments, which makes it easier for you to get sick – and stay sick. In contrast, when your body is more alkaline, bacteria and viruses are less able to survive and disease doesn't have as great of an opportunity to occur.

Finally, recognize that the impact of stress on your body is as powerful as the foods you eat. Any major stress will leave its acid residue. Because of the body's reaction to go into fight mode when stressed, excessive hormones are secreted and even foods that are alkaline will turn acidic.

Signs of an acid imbalance in your body:

- Weight gain, obesity and diabetes
- Lack of energy and constant fatigue
- Hormonal problems
- Osteoporosis and joint pain
- Slow digestion and elimination
- Headaches
- Tendency to get infections

Note that *gastric acid* (HCL) is an acid, but is vital for digestion. It allows the stomach to break food down and it maintains proper alkaline/acid balance. It becomes alkaline after its job is done. HCL is also our first line of defense against microbes that might enter our body with our food. Adequate HCL levels greatly decrease tissue acid waste build up.

Alkalinity

Alkaline imbalance is quite uncommon compared to acid imbalance. According to some authors, over-alkalinity is very rare and occurs in the blood, not in the tissues.

Alkaline-forming reaction refers to any changes in the body which produce an increased ability to energize the system and leaves an alkaline residue in the urine. Alkaline-forming minerals found in food are: calcium, magnesium, sodium, potassium, iron and manganese. When we ingest alkaline-forming minerals at one sitting, the remainder will be stored in the body tissues for future use.

PH of Common Foods

Ideally, you should be eating a diet consisting of at least a 60 percent of alkaline-forming foods and 40 percent acid-forming foods. And when you need to restore your health, the ratio should be more like 80 percent / 20 percent. Supplementing your diet by drinking blended green leafy vegetable drinks is a quick and easy way to create a more alkaline environment in your body (see chapter #18 – "Benefits Of Greens").

Below is a list of high acid-forming and high alkaline-forming foods. Some of the foods may surprise you. For example, a lemon is acidic to the taste but is actually alkaline forming in the body.

High Acidity

- Blueberries, cranberries, prunes and sweetened fruit juices
- Wheat, white bread, pastries, biscuits and pasta
- Beef, Pork and shellfish
- Cheese, homogenized milk, ice cream, custard
- Peanuts and walnuts
- Beer, liquor and soft drinks
- Artificial Sweeteners and chocolate

High Alkalinity

- Asparagus, onions, vegetable juices, parsley, raw spinach, broccoli, garlic, barley grass
- Lemon, watermelon, limes, grapefruit, mangoes, papayas
- Olive oil

- Herb Teas, lemon water
- Stevia

For a more complete list you can go online. You will be amazed at all the information available to you on the subject.

Ask Yourself...

- How can I create a healthy environment for my body?

- What am I putting into my body that might be setting it up for disease?

- What is my energy level throughout the day?

Your Wellness Strategies

- Go to your local health food store and buy pH strips. You will find two different types – one you can use with your saliva (might be more practical, but less reliable) and the other with your urine. Test your pH level in the morning and in the evening and compare with the desired pH levels discussed in this chapter.

- Today, write down everything you eat, assess each item's acidity or alkalinity using the information in this chapter and any information you gather online.

- Eliminate five acid-forming foods from your diet this week. Note how you feel and how your energy level changes.

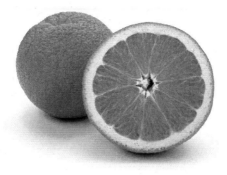

Chapter 18: Benefits Of Greens

– Dr. Nathalie

"He who has health, has hope; and he who has hope has everything."
– Arab Proverb

Due to our busy lifestyles, we don't always have the time or opportunity to eat properly. Coupled with a high quality multivitamin, you may want to consider adding a "green drink" as part of your daily supplement routine. Not to be confused with green tea, "green drinks" are a tremendous source of energy, help give your body a well-balanced pH by increasing your alkalinity, and provide the nutrients you may be missing from the meals void of green vegetables. Some "green drinks" are equivalent to five to six servings of organic fruits and vegetables!

Two kinds of green supplementation are readily available on the market: algae and cereal grass. The algae include chlorella, spirulina and green-blue algae. The grasses are wheat and barley grass.

Wheat Grass

Your health will profit greatly from wheat grass. Wheat grass' most important property lies in its 70 percent chlorophyll content.

The chlorophyll present in wheat grass helps the body by:

- Cleansing the bowel, liver and blood
- Aiding with digestion

- Deodorizing the body

- Promoting a healthy pH of the body

Wheat grass is also a rich source of natural vitamins, minerals and enzymes:

- Vitamins A, B, C and E

- Minerals – 92 of the 102 minerals available in the soil are absorbed by wheat grass including calcium, iron, sodium, potassium, and magnesium

- 17 amino acids – the building blocks of protein

- Rich in enzymes and will stimulate the body's own production of enzymes

And if that's not enough, wheat grass also stimulates the bowels to eliminate waste and supports thyroid functions.

Some "green drinks" on the market may substitute wheat grass with barley grass, which also has major health benefits. Barley grass is also rich in chlorophyll and fiber. It contains high amount of minerals, vitamins, amino acids and enzymes essential for healthy living.

It is important to note that wheat grass and barley grass do not contain gluten (see chapter #30 – "Gluten – Are You Sensitive To It?"). The grasses come from the powdered leaves of young plants *before* the grain stalk has started to develop. Gluten is later produced from the stalk and the head.

Other ingredients can be added to "green drinks" to enhance your energy level such as alfalfa, beet powders, bee pollen, royal jelly and liquorice. "Green drinks" shouldn't have any added sugar, artificial sweeteners or salt. Since "green drinks" come in powder form, some people mix it with juice or their favorite protein drink. Be aware however that not everyone can acquire a taste for "green drinks" – capsules are available for those who need an alternative.

Another benefit of most "green drinks" is that they contain essential ingredients including phytonutrients and fiber, making them a great whole food supplement.

Ask Yourself...

- Do I eat at least six servings of vegetables and fruits every day?

- Am I energetic throughout the day or do I tend to crash mid-day and reach for a coffee or sweets to revive myself?

- Do I suffer from chronic conditions like arthritis, irritable bowel syndrome or headaches? (These are indications that your body may be acidic and you could benefit from "green drinks").

- Do I eat enough alkalizing foods during the day to counteract a potentially acidic diet or lifestyle (stress)?.

Your Wellness Strategies

- Go to your favorite health food store or health care provider and determine which green supplement drink is best for you. Two of my favorite products are Greens + by Genuine Health and Nikken's organic Jade Greenzymes™.

- Simply put the green powder in a shaker cup and carry it with you on the go. Just add water and shake when you are ready to drink, wherever you are and whenever you need it!

- As an alternative, consider taking chlorella capsules or add liquid chlorophyll to your water (as per suggested serving on the bottle).

Note: Consult with your doctor before taking "green drinks" if you are taking medication.

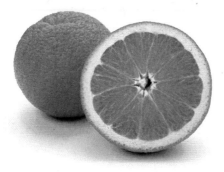

Chapter 19: Measure Up!

– Dr. Nathalie

"Our bodies communicate to us clearly and specifically, if we are willing to listen to them."

– Shakti Gawain

Body Mass Index, Waist to Hip Ratio, Body Fat Percentage

What do they all mean?

First, know that a healthy body is not defined by the number on the scale. We sometimes get too hung up on a number as opposed to taking a look at our overall health. A healthy weight range will only relate what is statistically considered for good health and decreased disease risk parameters. But weight alone is not a reliable indicator of good health.

There are several methods to determine what is a "healthy" weight and what is considered overweight and obese.

Body Mass Index (BMI)

BMI is one of the most common practical methods to determine healthy weight. It's easy to calculate, non-invasive, and has been proven to correlate well with health measures in population studies.

Method of Calculating BMI

The formula for calculating your BMI = Weight (kg)/Height (m)^2

- Convert your weight from pounds to kilograms by dividing by 2.2;

- Convert your height from feet to simply the number of inches (there are 12 inches in a foot);

- Convert your height from inches to meters by dividing by 39.4;

- Take your height in meters and square it by multiplying it by itself;

- Take your weight and divide it by your height in meters squared.

Example: 145 lbs ÷ 2.2 = 65.9 kg

       5 feet 9 = 12 x 5 + 9 = 69 inches

       69 inches ÷ 39.4 = 1.75 meters

       $(1.75 \text{ meters})^2 = 3.06$ meters squared

       65.9 kg ÷ 3.06 meters squared = 21.5 body mass index

BMI – Body Mass Index Interpretation

Canadian BMI Guidelines

- Underweight = <20.0
- Healthy weight = 20-25
- Overweight = 25-27
- Obesity = BMI of 27 or greater

U.S. BMI Guidelines

- Underweight = <18.5
- Healthy weight = 18.5-24.9
- Overweight = 25-29.9
- Obesity = BMI of 30 or greater

Note – BMI parameters seem to change depending on the different sources. Canada and U.S. parameters also seem to differ slightly.

If you don't feel like calculating your own BMI, just log onto the Internet and type in body mass index. There are a multitude of sites that will do the calculations for you.

BMI numbers are guidelines but they aren't perfect. A body builder for example may not have a good BMI, so taking a body fat percentage test in this case would be a better indicator. Calculating BMI for children or adolescents is not recommended due to growth spurts which cause fluctuations in weight.

Waist to Hip Ratio (WHR)

We all carry our weight differently, some people carry excess weight in the abdomen area and others in the lower portion of the body. The Waist to Hip Ratio measurement will help determine where you store your fat. If you carry a lot of your weight in the abdominal region, your risk of disease increases because of the proximity of the fat to the organs in the area; pancreas, liver, and heart.

The formula for your Waist to Hip Ratio (WHR) = waist in centimeters ÷ by hips in centimeters

If your result is greater than 1.0 (for men) or 0.8 (for women), you have a greater risk of health problems; particularly cardiovascular diseases like heart attack, diabetes and high blood pressure.

Waist to Hip Ratio Interpretation

	Excellent	Good	Average	High	Extreme
Male	≤ 0.85	0.85- 0.90	0.90 – 0.95	0.95 – 1.00	≥ 1.00
Female	≤ 0.75	0.75- 0.80	0.80 – 0.85	0.85 – 0.90	≥ 0.90

Body Fat Measurements

Why measure body fat? The main reason is to determine whether you have a healthy body weight or whether you're at risk for weight-related diseases. Measuring your body fat will also help you evaluate the success of your current nutrition and exercise program.

Since your weight on the scale doesn't take into account your lean muscle mass, measuring body fat will give you a better idea of how much weight you need to lose, fat weight, not muscle weight. Our metabolic rate plays a crucial role in our efficiency to burn calories. The higher the lean muscle mass, the higher the metabolic rate making the body more efficient at burning calories. Do keep in mind that a certain amount of fat is essential for the body to function. Fat regulates body temperature, cushions and insulates organs and tissues and is the main form of the body's energy storage.

Methods of Measuring Body Fat

- *DEXA* – stands for Dual Energy X-Ray Absorptiometry. Low level X-Rays at two different energy levels are used to determine body composition. Highly accurate but expensive and inconvenient. Considered the "gold standard" for body fat measurements.

- *Underwater Weighing in a Water Tank* – a highly accurate method to determine the percentage of body fat but not very common or practical.

- *Bioelectrical Impedance Analysis* – An unnoticeable electrical current passes though the body to estimate how much water the body contains, which reflects the amount of lean tissue. Over or under hydration can result in inaccurate readings. This form of measurement also requires adherence to a strict testing protocol, including fasting and voiding the bowel – which many people ignore. Therefore, results are often imprecise.

- *Near Infrared Light* – This measurement method can be done in a matter of seconds. Infrared light is used at specific frequencies. The difference between the amount of light absorbed versus the amount of light reflected is measured to calculate the percentage of fat. This is a very non-invasive and fairly precise method of measuring body fat (unless the person is severely underweight or overweight).

- *Skin Fold Thickness* – This is the most common and inexpensive way to measure body fat. Calipers are used to measure the thickness of skin folds. Measurements are taken at specific areas of the body. Reliability is questionable as the method used may vary from one examiner to another.

Body Fat Percentage

Age of adult female	Increased disease risk	Healthy	Increased disease risk	Greatly increased disease risk
20 to 39	0 to 21%	21% to 33%	33% to 39%	39% and above
40 to 59	0 to 23%	23% to 34%	34% to 40%	40% and above
60 to 79	0 to 24%	24% to 36%	36% to 42%	42% and above

Age of adult male	Increased disease risk	Healthy	Increased disease risk	Greatly increased disease risk
20 to 39	0 to 8%	8% to 20%	20% to 25%	25% and above
40 to 59	0 to 11%	11% to 22%	22% to 28%	28% and above
60 to 79	0 to 13%	13% to 25%	25% to 30%	30% and above

Ask Yourself...

- Do I know my Body Mass Index (BMI) score, Waist to Hip Ratio (WHR) score or body fat percentage?

- Where can I go to get my body fat measured accurately?

- Do any of my scores indicate a health risk?

Your Wellness Strategies

- Calculate your Body Mass Index (BMI) and Waist to Hip Ratio (WHR);

- If your scores are a health risk, make an appointment with your Wellness Team to determine the best strategy to make the changes required. Don't wait!

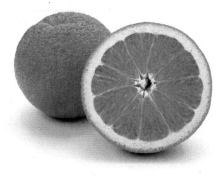

Chapter 20: The Little Voice Inside Your Head

– Andrée

"All talking, all thinking, all thoughts must be pure."

– Yogi Bhajan

A coaching client invited me to the opening of his and his wife's new business. When I arrived I was greeted by the proud owners and given a tour of their store. It was everything they had worked for, they said. I was introduced to other guests by my client as "a friend and my coach." He mentioned to the guests that I had coached him for a year and that this business was the culmination of his coaching process. Imagine that! "Wow" I thought to myself, "How great is that?" I felt really good, knowing that in some way I had been instrumental in helping this couple achieve their dream. When I left the store, I must tell you that I felt just a little envious. For as long as I can remember, I had wanted my own business, my own store. And here I was facing the undeniable fact that my coaching had assisted this couple in reaching their goal. Why was that not happening to me? Why was I not reaching all my goals?

As I looked back over a successful career, I realized that throughout my life I have helped hundreds of people reach beyond themselves. As a manager, I have helped people get promotions, change jobs and become very successful in various organizations. As a coach, I have helped people start new careers, open businesses, build existing businesses to award-winning success and build individual self-confidence so that they could become who they really wanted to be. Obviously I was saying something to these people that was compelling them to reach greater heights. I was somehow helping them manifest their inner most dreams. And, while at that stage of my life, I could say that I owned my own business, I was struggling emotionally and financially.

So in early morning meditation, I started asking the coach inside of me to help me become everything I wanted to be. I started doing as my employees and clients did – I started listening to the voice inside of me. What was it saying? Was it uplifting, encouraging and motivating? Was the voice asking me to be accountable? Or was it telling me to deny my true self; the self that wanted the lake house as a peaceful retreat, the self that wanted to be an international motivational speaker who could reach hundreds of people at a time? I guess I always heard a negative voice inside but never paid much attention. It had become such a pattern to listen to the negative thoughts, the disparaging, downplaying voice that said "…that's not for you" or "you're not good enough" or "you're from the wrong side of the tracks, so you have to be happy with less."

All in all, on the outside, my friends thought I was successful and thought I was a very positive person. I had a house, a healthy and well-balanced teenage son and close supportive friends, yet there was always something beyond my reach. My finances were worse than my relationships, one minute I would have money, the next I didn't. I was on a virtual roller coaster ride. What was I doing wrong?

You see the obvious disconnect? On the one hand, I was encouraging and motivating clients and, in the same breath, I was discouraging and putting myself down. The more I concentrated on my inner voice, the more it became clear to me that I was programmed to sabotage myself. My inner voice, like a computer program, had a virus and it was infecting all of my positive files. Every time I tried to change the program outwardly, like getting into a new relationship or losing weight, the new program would work for a little while and then the virus would rapidly worm its way into the new file and zap, I was right back where I started.

Like anything else, if you don't know what is wrong you can't fix it! As Dr. Nathalie mentions in her chapter about listening to your body, you must first hear it and feel it before you can change it. In my process of discovery, I started listening, really listening to the little voice inside my head. I noticed for example that when I woke up one of the first thoughts in my head was that I was fat. I would say things to myself like "I ate too much yesterday, my stomach is huge" or "Oh God, what if I can't pay those bills?" "What if I lose my job?" or "I'm so tired. I am so old" These were the first thoughts in my head – great way to start the day, right? I was so programmed; I don't think I really noticed until I started listening. I wanted to give myself the gift of what I was giving my clients, of what I had given my staff and the only way to do that was to listen to myself. Now that I knew that the thoughts were, shall we say, less than encouraging, I could start changing the programming. One step at a time, one day at a time.

Does any of this sound familiar to you? Have you experienced this in your own life? Are you the type of person who can encourage others, help others in boosting their self-esteem and yet you can't seem to do it for yourself? What is your inner voice telling you? How can you start listening? How can you decipher what your internal programming is? A good place to start is with simple things.

Have you ever heard your little voice saying: "Don't eat that cookie!" or "Those fries smell great but you promised yourself not to eat so many fatty foods!" And then, of course, there is the other voice that says, "Go ahead, what difference will one cookie make?" or "You deserve those fries. You've had a hard day at work." We've all had mornings when we've set our alarms for 5:30 a.m. with the best intention of getting up to exercise, but when the alarm goes off a little voice whispers "Don't bother. It's so cold outside and this bed is so comfortable. Just press the snooze button and sleep in a little more."

What is your programmed mind telling you to do? Will you go for the cookie or eat those fries? Stop yourself and listen carefully. Be mindful of your goal and your dream. Do you start your day by thinking negative thoughts about yourself and the way you live your life? What you *should* or *should not* be doing that day? That little voice inside your head telling you all those negative things make you feel so unworthy of changing. Maybe, you even tell yourself, "What does it matter if I miss my exercise routine? I'm overweight anyway" or "What difference will it make if I miss yoga today? It's not important."

If your goal is to be at your optimal weight and feel healthy and energetic, yet you indulge in too many snacks and don't exercise, what is your pre-programmed mind telling you? Who are you letting down? If you were encouraging a friend who wants to get fit, what would you tell her? What could you be telling yourself? How can you take corrective action? Your inner voice guides you in your decisions every day. These decisions then map the course of your actions and affect your present and future.

Motivational speaker, Loretta Laroche, revealed in her seminar "The Joy of Stress" that appeared on PBS a number of years ago, that 75 percent of our daily conversations are negative. Is it any wonder we feel so crappy a lot of the time or that we can't reach our goals?

I believe that deep down inside of us there is that positive voice, that healthy program to tell us we can live our dreams and reach our goals. I believe we truly deserve to live a happy, healthy life. I also believe that we somehow, like a computer program, over time, have been infected with a negative thought virus and it has corrupted our positive thought files. A baby learning to walk is symbolic of what we, as human beings, can truly achieve. Imagine the strength and determination it takes for a baby to first crawl, then stand, and of course, fall and fall again. Yet they never stop for one moment and think, "I can't do this, I will never walk." When the baby falls, he will stand up, find support, and try again and again. As parents, we encourage, we smile, we hold, we reach out to baby, validating the efforts and the success. We need to relearn to do that for ourselves. We need to become our own coach; encouraging, nurturing, smiling, and reaching out with approval.

You already are everything you can be…somewhere inside. It's all there waiting for you to listen, waiting for you to believe and to take corrective actions where necessary.

Listen…can you hear the applause?

ASK YOURSELF…

- What is my inner voice telling me today?

- What changes can I make today to replace my negative thoughts?

- What food choices can I make today to follow my positive inner voice?

YOUR WELLNESS STRATEGIES

- Take time to notice your positive inner voice. Write in your journal the choices you made that were guided by that positive inner voice.

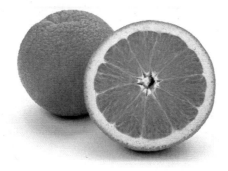

Chapter 21: Cardiovascular Training –
The Heart Of The Matter

– Dr. Nathalie

"Fitness – If it came in a bottle, everybody would have a great body."
– Cher

There are so many different schools of thought when it comes to exercising your heart and lungs. Experts' opinion on cardiovascular training varies on: the length of time one should exercise, the intensity and even the types of exercise. The goal of this chapter is to make you think about the effectiveness of the way you exercise so that you can get the most out of your work-out. Remember, there are different roads to achieve your fitness goals but as the popular tag line would have it, "Just do it!"

Benefits of a Cardiovascular Workout

- Improved cardiovascular and respiratory functions;

- Decreased resting heart rate and blood pressure;

- Decreased risks of death from coronary artery disease;

- Decreased anxiety and depression;

- Enhanced physical ability and independent-living in older persons;

- Enhanced feeling of well-being;

- Enhanced performance at work and recreational/sport activities;

- Reduced unhealthy weight gain;

- Lowered incidence of cardiovascular disease, stroke, Type 2 Diabetes, osteoporosis, colon cancer, breast cancer and gallbladder disease.

My Personal Quest for the "Right" Workout

The main goal with cardiovascular exercise is to keep your heart and lungs in tip-top shape, but for most people it also means keeping their body lean and maintaining a healthy weight. Having a bachelor's degree in human kinetics, I was always fascinated by the topic of how one could best achieve and maintain fitness goals. It always puzzled me that some aerobic instructors or marathon runners, who seemed to be in great shape, were often overweight and seemed to have lower muscle mass. It just didn't add up! How can these people exercise so much and still be overweight? Over the years, I have experimented with several approaches to exercise for myself to evaluate the different results.

Here is my story! Years of natural bodybuilding with little "cardio" and a lot of "heavy" weights allowed me to stay fairly lean and maintain a good muscle mass. Last year, I wanted to try something different and decided to run my first marathon (I know, most people would have started with a 10 km or a half marathon – I went for the full deal – that is just me!). It was a great experience all around but I noticed two major things. While I was training for my marathon, I really decreased my weight training to accommodate the time spent running. I started noticing changes in my body. I was losing muscle mass and gaining fat (my body fat percentage was increasing), even though I was technically spending a lot more calories. What was happening? I also noticed that my lung capacity had decreased. One would expect it to increase while training for a marathon. How could that be? This might explain why an endurance athlete can succumb to a heart attack at rest! Heart attacks don't happen due to a lack of endurance, but often because of a sudden increase in cardiac demand exceeding your heart's capacity.

My experiment had given me two revelations: long distance running does not necessarily mean lower body fat or better lung capacity. Yes, the heart and lungs need to be stressed to increase or preserve their capacities, but that does not necessarily mean long endurance sessions are the answer. Think about it – how often does one get chased by a bear for 26 miles?

My point here is that if we look at our ancestors, obesity was almost non-existent and nobody really "exercised". What was most needed back then, were short bursts of exercise to stay clear of dangerous situations or to hunt for food. Long duration exercise equals prolonged stress on the body. Actually, studies have shown signs of heart distress, increased low density lipoprotein (LDL), increased triglycerides (TG), increased oxidation of cholesterol, elevated clotting and inflammation factors and a loss of bone density. Now you're thinking, "Great, I don't have to exercise!" That is not what I'm saying! You need to exercise, but you need to be smart about it.

Read on... you will love this! You may not need to exercise as long as you think! I recently came across the work of Dr. Al Sears who has been in the field of exercise for over 25 years. His PACE™ training method is based on the theory that continuous, endurance exercise actually induces your heart and lungs to "downsize" as the body adapts to the demand. The PACE™ system is designed to challenge peak lung volume. When you exercise "above" your aerobic zone (what he calls your supra-aerobic zone – high output and short duration) you create an oxygen debt sending signals to your lungs to expand. In turn, this forces your lungs to adapt by increasing their volume and power as well as building your heart reserve capacity. Your reserve capacity means your heart has the ability to pump more blood, faster in times of stress. For your lungs, it means they are able to deal with high exertion activities like lifting or running for the bus. Without a good reserve capacity, you are more likely to have a detrimental reaction to a high stress situation. Exercising in this supra-aerobic zone, according to Dr. Sears, can also help you burn fat more efficiently and decrease its storage.

Typically, what most of us have learned through the years is that you need to be in a certain intensity or "zone" to burn fat. Below is a chart showing the percentages of protein, carbohydrates and fat our bodies use as "fuel" when performing activities at different intensity.

Activity level	Protein	Carbs	Fat
Resting	1 to 5%	35%	60%
Low intensity	5-8%	70%	15%
Moderate Intensity	2-5%	40%	55%
High Intensity	2%	95%	3%

This chart is still true today, but the important question remains, is using fat as our principal fuel the best way to stay lean? Your body's adaptation will be to store more fat to better prepare for the next time you exercise and by doing so, it most likely will sacrifice muscles. Your body will be saying: "food – I better store that as fat, because we are going to be running for a long time again tomorrow." This defeats the purpose, doesn't it? According to the above mentioned chart, why not just rest and burn more calories from fat!?

Dr. Sears emphasizes that the way you exercise will affect the way your metabolism operates for the next few days facilitating fat burning. He suggests short-burst exercises that will tell your body not to store fat as energy because it will not be using it. You will use carbohydrates for the exercise and burn the fat after your exercise session is done. Several studies were done comparing short-burst training versus long-term endurance training. Results show an increase in muscle mass and a decrease in fat percentage with the short burst training. This really makes sense to me and would explain why body builders and sprinters are so muscular and lean.

Here are some of the benefits of short-burst exercises on your health, it will:

- Improve maximum cardiac output
- Better cardiac adjustment to your heart's demand
- Help your body lose fat in as little as 10 minutes per day
- Improve cholesterol levels
- Provide some anti-aging benefits

My first thought when reading about this was, "Brilliant, but what about the person who is really out of shape – aren't they going to hurt themselves?" Your higher intensity level is uniquely yours and you don't have to start by sprinting down the street full throttle from the get-go! An elliptical or a recumbent bike can safely do the job. Always with any exercise program, please consult your doctor.

Getting to Know Your Heart Rate at Rest and During Exercise

You will often see at the gym, colored charts to guide you, but those charts only take into consideration a person's age and not their level of fitness. A 40-year old marathon runner's fitness condition will be very different than a 40-year-old who never exercises. This is why one's resting heart rate needs to be taken into the equation to truly evaluate one's working "zone". To find your individual "zone," take your resting heart rate when you wake up in the morning, before you do anything else. To do this, take your right index and middle finger and put them on the inside of your wrist close to your thumb and count the beats for 15 seconds. Then multiply that number by four to calculate your one-minute count.

Next, with your resting heart rate, calculate your optimal cardiovascular range using the heart rate reserve method:

Target heart rate lower limit =   (220 – age) – Resting Heart Rate x
0.60 + Resting Heart Rate

Target heart rate upper limit =   (220 – age) – Resting Heart Rate x
0.80 + Resting Heart Rate

For example:

My morning resting heart rate is 50 and I'm 39 years old:

(220 – 39) – 50 x 0.60 +50 =   129 beats per minute is the lower limit
of workout range .

(220 – 39) – 50 x 0.80 +50 =   155 beats per minute is the higher limit
of workout range

My exercise zone should be between 129 and 155 beats per minute. When working with short-burst exercise, I should be working at the upper end of that zone or even a little higher.

Tools to Help You

Heart rate monitors are readily available to help you measure your heart rate and stay within your zone. This eliminates the trouble of counting your heart beats per minute, which can sometimes be challenging when you are exercising. It will also help you record your workout and keep you on track with your goals. You can buy them at any sporting goods stores.

You can find out more information on the PACE™ program at www.alsears. com. You can order his book, where he gives you the necessary steps to customize your own program and achieve amazing results.

One of my favorite fast and convenient routines is the skipping rope. One minute jumping plus one minute rest for 10 times, equals a 20-minute workout in total. I keep track of my heart rate at the end of the minute and just before starting to jump again. My chart looks something like this:

	Heart rate after 1 minute of jumping	Heart rate after 1 minute of rest
1	139	73
2	144	71
3	140	65
4	136	72
5	148	76
6	152	83
7	158	86
8	152	80
9	156	85
10	153	79

You can perform interval training on the bike or the elliptical. Now, this does not mean you should not run a marathon if you truly enjoy it! This information is a guide to give you another way to look at your exercise program. Exercise on the go...means short and efficient workouts that will help you reap the best benefits!

ASK YOURSELF...

- Do I know my resting heart rate and my optimal cardiovascular zone?

- Do I use my heart rate to monitor the efficiency of my work-outs?

- Am I willing to try interval training to maximize my workout results?

Your Wellness Strategies

- Buy a heart monitor and calculate your resting heart rate and your optimal cardiovascular zone.

- Design yourself an interval training program (e.g. skipping rope, biking or running) or find a program that works for you.

- Record your heart rate at the beginning and the end of each interval – monitor your recovery time.

- Remember to start slowly! Consult with your doctor or a qualified health care professional before starting any physical program.

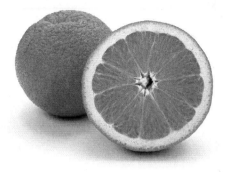

Chapter 22: Strength Training – "Tour De Force"

– Dr. Nathalie

"Never eat more than you can lift."
– Miss Piggy, Muppet Show

When it comes to exercise and getting fit, most women think about cardio first. Go to any gym and you'll see most of the women sweating it out on cardio equipment – the treadmills, elliptical machines, bikes – while most men are in the weight room area. As women, we need to change our perception about exercise. While cardio *is* necessary to obtain and maintain good physical condition and overall health, strength training is just as important for total well-being.

So often I hear women say they don't want to try strength training because they don't want to get big and "bulky" like Arnold Schwarzenegger. The good news is it just won't happen – women don't have the testosterone levels required to get that big!

One of the many advantages of strength training is that it increases lean muscle mass. A greater lean muscle mass positively impacts the efficiency of our metabolism to burn calories. Here is the example I often give: two women weigh 150 pounds; one has 36 percent body fat and 98 pounds of muscle, the other has 22 percent body fat and 118 pounds of muscle. The one with the higher muscle mass will burn more calories. So even though the two women are the same weight, the one with the higher muscle mass will be able to have a higher caloric intake than the other woman while maintaining her weight. How great is that! But there's more to it ...strength training is empowering; it feels good to be strong!

Benefits of Strength Training

- Increases strength of muscles, tendons and ligaments
- Increases stability of joints
- Increases muscle mass
- Increases bone density and bone mass
- Improves body composition
- Improves motor coordination
- Reduces the risk of osteoporosis
- Reduces the signs and symptoms of chronic diseases such as Arthritis and Type 2 Diabetes
- Improves sleep and reduces sleep disorders
- Reduces depression
- Improves flexibility
- Reduces the number of falls in older adults
- Reduces severity of injuries by strengthening supportive structures, developing muscle balance around joints and increasing your muscles' ability to absorb energy

Free-Weights vs. Machines

Strength training with free-weights, when done properly and with good form is generally more beneficial than training with machines. This is primarily because most machines can't be adjusted perfectly for your size. This can cause you to a) do the exercise wrong; b) do it in a way that hurts you; and c) do it in a way that doesn't benefit you. The range of motion is also more limited on machines. In comparison, the range of motion with free weights resembles the movements you do in everyday life: this will benefit you more. Still, there is controversy and disagreement over which is better; some personal trainers prefer machines as a safer alternative when clients aren't used to lifting weights.

Free-Weight Pros

- Increases the use of your stabilizing muscles, thereby increasing your core strength
- The range of motion when using free-weights is similar to everyday activities
- Hones your perception of balance and the location of your body in the space around you
- It's convenient and inexpensive!

Free-Weight Cons

- Increases risk of injury if you don't use proper form
- You spend a lot of time changing weights
- If your gym doesn't have a lot of free-weights, you may spend a lot of time waiting for the ones you want

Machine Pros

- Can be great for beginners
- Offers an array of weight choices
- Can prevent some injuries since the machines control the range of motion
- Faster workouts – easier transition from one machine to another

Machine Cons

- Increases the risk of overuse and injuries
- Mistaken sense of safety – you can overload your muscles with too much weight
- Locks your body in place with specific movement patterns – with free weights you can respect the body's natural range of motion

Dr. Nathalie's 19 Tips for Optimal Strength Training Success

1. <u>Hire a trainer</u> – it's worth the money, especially if you're not comfortable or familiar with strength training;

2. <u>Warm up</u> – strength training is a high-effort physical activity. It is crucial that you warm up by increasing your body temperature

(for example – by walking on the treadmill for five to 10 minutes) and do some activity that allows you to get your body warmed in preparation for your weight training;

3. Stretching – perform light stretching of the muscle group you will be working on to warm up the muscles and surrounding joints. It is important that you do not stretch too much as it can be detrimental to proper muscle contraction. A good way to warm up is by performing the specific exercise you plan to do with very light weights;

4. Technique – above all, remember that good technique is crucial to your progress and to prevent injuries. When weight training is done right, there should not be any injuries. Aim for the right form using the proper weight;

5. Angle – one important strategy with weight training is to be able to work your muscles at different angles to stimulate muscle growth and balance the development of the muscle. For example, the pectoral muscle (chest muscle) can be worked at three different angles: a) you can work the top part of the muscle with an incline bench (bench at a 45-degree incline); b) you can work the more central part of the muscle with a flat bench; c) you can work the lower part of the pectoral muscle with a decline bench. These three different exercises will fully challenge the different muscle fibers;

6. Tempo – tempo is another very important variation you can make in your workouts to challenge your muscles in different ways. For example, a "5-2-5" tempo for bench press means you push for the count of five seconds, hold for two seconds and lower for the count of five again. You will be amazed at how much harder it makes lifting the weight! It's a great way to challenge your muscles differently;

7. Resistance – remember that strength training is also called "resistance training" and for good reason. If you can complete a set of 25 repetitions, you're not using enough weight, and you're not creating enough resistance for your muscles. For strength training to be beneficial, you actually need to create micro tears in your muscles, which will trigger them to "self-repair," which is what makes them grow stronger;

8. Repetitions and sets – repetitions are the number of times you do a movement with a weight, while sets are how many times you

do those repetitions. Sets of 12 repetitions are the most common but you can do drop-sets by decreasing the number of repetitions with each set, while increasing the weight. For example, you could do 12 bicep curls with a 10-pound dumbbell on the first set, 10 bicep curls with a 12-pound dumbbell on the second, and eight bicep curls with a 15-pound dumbbell on the third. By doing drop-sets, you will fully challenge your biceps, and leave them close to exhaustion. Also, for optimal results, it's important to alter the sets and repetitions because muscles have memory and they will quickly adapt to your routine, which will slow your progress (plateau);

9. Super-sets or giant-sets – if you're in a hurry or want to try something quick and different, do super-sets or giant-sets. A super-set consists of two exercises alternated twice without rest. For example, when working your chest you could do a set of bench presses, followed by a set of push ups; then repeat. For your giant-set, which consists of three exercises done three times without rest, you could add sets of cable flies (in a circuit format);

10. Concentric exercises versus eccentric exercises – concentric exercises shorten your muscles while eccentric exercises elongate your muscles. Both are important. The preacher curl is a good example of an eccentric exercise because it stretches the biceps to its full length in the down position. A good example of a concentric exercise is the concentrated bicep curl, where the muscle remains contracted for most of the exercise. It's important to have a mix of the two types of exercises in your workouts to effectively maximize the challenge to your muscles. I strongly suggest that you start with the eccentric exercises in order to engage the muscle through its entire range and then move on to concentric ones;

11. Cable exercises – these are good to incorporate into your workout. You can use cables in lieu of dumbbells or barbells, since these offer consistent tension throughout the movement and also increase the use of surrounding stabilizing muscles;

12. Unilateral and bilateral exercises – in a unilateral exercise, you use one side at a time during strength training, while in a bilateral exercise you use both sides. Since most people have a dominant side, it's important to integrate both types in order to balance your musculature, and to effectively use your core muscles;

13. <u>Variation of exercises</u> – it's crucial to alter your workout regularly. Some people do the same things at the gym for years and wonder why they don't see the results they want. As I mentioned earlier, muscles adapt quickly, so you need to keep finding new ways of challenging them – even just to maintain your current muscle tone. I know – it sounds complicated. But it also keeps you from getting bored or staying at a plateau;

14. <u>Breathe</u> – don't forget to breathe! Exhale during more demanding concentric muscle movements (concentric exercises are ones that will shorten your muscle) and you'll prevent excessive internal pressure that restricts blood flow back to the heart that could make you lightheaded or dizzy;

15. <u>Length of workout</u> – your strength training workout shouldn't exceed one hour. If you strength train for longer than that, you have a greater chance of getting injured and your muscles will be too tired or depleted to be productive;

16. <u>Cool down</u> – this is very important as it helps your muscular system and cardiovascular system return to a resting state. Five to ten minutes on a stationary bike, for example, is a good way to cool down. You should do most of your stretching in the cool-down phase and focus particularly on the body parts you have worked that day;

17. <u>Recuperation</u> – you need to give your muscles time to recuperate and regenerate. As mentioned earlier, when you train with weights, you actually create micro-tears in your muscles which, when given the time to heal, will repair and grow stronger. If you don't give your body the time to regenerate, these muscles lose some of the benefits of strength training. Too many people do too much and then get discouraged when they get injured. Sometimes less is more!;

18. <u>Fitness Journal</u> – I know…groan! But a log book helps you keep your commitment to your fitness and measures your improvement. Keeping track of the weight you use allows you to always be ready, saves you time and pushes you to the next level;

19. <u>Have fun!</u> Hundreds of great different and varied workout examples are out there! The key is to change it up and have fun with them. Add variation to your routine, otherwise your body will adapt, which will slow your progress and diminish your results.

Dr. Nathalie's 4-day Workout

One of the strength training workouts I really like involves four days a week and two major body parts per workout! You can opt to do cardio on the other days or even on the same day, if you have time (no more than 30 minutes). I always try adding one or two core muscle group exercises (working the abdominal and stabilizing muscles) towards the end of my workout. Below is an example of one of my strength training workouts. You'll need the use of a full gym to do this but you can always modify some of the exercises if you're working out at home. For more information on this workout or other workouts, visit www.drnathaliebeauchamp.ca.

Day 1 – Chest, Biceps and Core

1) Flat bench press with barbell

2) Bicep preacher curl with EZ bar

3) Incline bench press with dumbbell

4) Bicep hammer curl

5) Decline bench fly

6) Bicep concentrated curl with dumbbell

7) Push-up on exercise ball

8) Side plank on floor

Day 2 – Back, Triceps and Core

1) Back pull-down with wide grip bar

2) Barbell triceps extension skull-crusher with the EZ bar

3) Bent-over row on bench

4) Cable triceps extension

5) Seated cable row with narrow grip

6) Triceps kickback

7) "Superperson" exercise on ball

8) Front plank

Day 3 – Legs and Core

1) Squat

2) Stiff leg dead lift

3) Lunge with dumbbell

4) Bench step-up with dumbbell

5) Machine leg extension

6) Sumo squat with dumbbell

7) Machine leg curl

8) Exercise ball hamstring curl

9) Hanging leg-raise

10) Ball crunch

Day 4 – Trapezius Muscles, Shoulders, Calves and Core

1) Standing barbell shrug

2) Standing barbell shoulder press

3) Standing calf raise

4) Shoulder side lateral raise

5) Shoulder front raise

6) Seated calf raise

7) Reverse fly- dumbbell on the ball

8) Rotator cuff on the ball

9) Cable crunch

10) Abs-ball leg tuck

ASK YOURSELF…

- Am I using strength training as part of my normal exercise regime?

- Do I understand the physical benefits of weight training?

- Am I intimidated by the weights or the people in the weight room?

- Do I need a trainer to help me with my strength training goals?

YOUR WELLNESS STRATEGIES

- Try the above workout or hire a qualified personal trainer to set up a customized program that will suit your needs.

- Buy a logbook to record and monitor your strength training progress.

- Set yourself monthly goals that include what you want to achieve physically.

- Find a training partner who will help you obtain your goals and keep it fun!

Note: Before you attempt any exercise program, please check with your doctor.

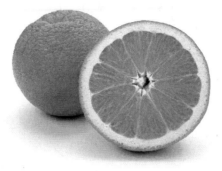

Chapter 23: Pump Up Your Self Confidence

– Andrée

"Let me pump you up!"
– Arnold Schwarzenegger

Think of a time when you felt absolutely fantastic about a project you completed, a task you did, a new skill you learned or a goal that you met. Can you remember that feeling? That excitement? What did it make you want to do? Tell everyone about it? Or maybe you wanted to start another project right away because you felt confident that you could do it all over again? Herein lies the operative word…you felt confident!

Self-confidence is the belief that we have the ability to succeed. It is also, knowing who we are and what we are capable of doing. When our self-confidence is high, we notice that people treat us differently; they may compliment us on how we look, or behave in a different manner, perhaps more positively or with more respect.

Also, when our self-confidence is pumped up, what people say about us, and other people's views about us will be of less concern – it won't affect us as much because we know we are great. On the other hand, if our self-confidence is low, any type of criticism can throw us off, take our focus away from our day and, in extreme cases, even make us feel depressed.

Remember: "You are what you think." Be aware of, and listen to, your inner dialogue. Have you ever noticed what you say to yourself in the morning when you first look in the mirror? Does the monologue go something like this: "Man I want to go back to bed. Look how puffy my eyes are. I really need to lose a few pounds. And look at those wrinkles." Or: "I hate it when I do that. I'll never be good enough so why even try?" Sound familiar? If your inner dialogue is anything like this, you're most likely suffering from low "confidenceitis."

The fact of the matter is that our inner dialogue – our inner thought process is actually controlling our lives. It controls how we interact with others, how we sell ourselves at work, how we present ourselves in relationships and how we treat ourselves. Ultimately, how we think of ourselves and how we talk to ourselves will directly affect our success in everything we do. The scariest part of this equation is that many of us are completely unaware of our own negative thoughts.

Weightlifting for Bulkier Self-Confidence

The first step to becoming more self-confident is becoming aware of the way we treat ourselves. It starts with listening and observing how we think, how we act and what we say to ourselves.

Once you've observed your inner dialogue and thought process, and you realize the negative impact it has on your life, you are ready to make life-changing choices. So get ready. This is a powerful exercise; you might be surprised by what you're actually telling yourself every day, maybe even several times a day.

ASK YOURSELF ... #1

Go to a place where you will feel comfortable and will be undisturbed, take your journal out and write down the answers to the following questions:

- What do I tell myself, about myself, every day?

- What are some of the words I use to describe myself?

- How do those words make me feel?

Your Wellness Strategies #1

- When you're done, find a mirror, look right in it, smile and say "Helloooo, handsome/gorgeous. You sure look great today." Add something like: "You really did a good job today at work," or "That meal you made tonight was such a success." Tell yourself how wonderful you are in10 different ways. It'll make you smile.

- Notice the difference in your face when you smile instead of frown. Notice how you feel when you use positive language about yourself.

Ask Yourself ... #2

- What am I most proud of in my life?

- What have I accomplished that I feel good about?

Your Wellness Strategies #2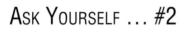

Many people forget about everything they've accomplished in life and compare themselves to others, thinking that others have accomplished so much more. This minimizes their self-confidence. This exercise will help combat the effects of "minimil*itis*" and will really pump up your self confidence.

Return to your journal and your special area. In your journal, list all that you have achieved or accomplished so far in your life. At first, it may appear to be a difficult exercise but as you get going, it will become lighter and easier. You have accomplished a lot so just let your thoughts flow. Write at least 20 items on your list. Here is a sample list:

- I finished high school

- I was the first one to go to university in my family

YOUR WELLNESS STRATEGIES #2 (CONT)

- I own a house/condo
- I own a car
- I have a good job or own a business
- I raised wonderful kids
- I exercise regularly
- I am constantly on a quest for self-improvement and look after myself (e.g. reading this book)
- I cook nourishing and delicious meals

Re-read your accomplishment list daily and continue to build on it

ASK YOURSELF ... #3

Starting your day with an attitude of gratitude is a sure way to put a spring in your step and a smile on your face, adding muscle to your confidence.

In the morning, take out your journal and go to your favorite chair. Sit comfortably and ask yourself the following questions, writing down at least 10 answers.

- What am I grateful for in my life?
- What am I grateful for about myself?
- What am I grateful for in my surroundings?

YOUR WELLNESS STRATEGIES #3

- Write down 10 new things you're grateful for every day for 21 days.
- Have fun, enjoy and watch your self-confidence muscles start to grow!!!

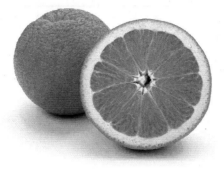

Chapter 24: Yoga For Your Body, Mind And Soul

– Andrée

"Yoga is the perfect opportunity to be curious about who you are."
– Jason Crandell

We have introduced you to various types of exercise – core strength, aerobic and weight-bearing. But exercising options would not be complete without talking about yoga.

Yoga is a form of exercise that affects all dimensions of you as a person: mind, body and soul. With yoga, every part of the body is treated with care and respect because there's recognition that it's the primary instrument for living well.

Yoga is derived from an ancient Indian body of knowledge that dates back more than 5,000 years. The word "yoga" comes from the Sanskrit word "yuj" meaning "to unite or integrate." Yoga is about integrating your own consciousness with the universal consciousness around you.

Ancient Yogis had a belief that for humans to be in harmony and balance with themselves and with their environment, they had to integrate their body, mind and spirit. For these three things to be integrated, however, emotion, action, and intelligence must be balanced. The Yogis formulated a way to achieve and maintain this balance, through exercise, breathing and meditation.

What Yoga Can Do For You

Unlike some exercises that require certain skills, yoga is for anyone with a willingness to learn. It doesn't require any special equipment, clothing or physical condition; it just requires the determination to achieve a healthier, stress-free self. In fact, you can even practice some forms of yoga if you are bedridden or wheelchair-bound.

Yoga can benefit your mind and body in a variety of ways. Physically, it improves circulation, oxygenates the blood, stimulates all organs, expands lung capacity and regulates the glandular system in the body, resulting in better health.

Certain styles of yoga, like Kundalini yoga, focus on balancing the body, mind and spirit, while other styles focus more on the physical benefits of the movements and poses of yoga.

Styles of Yoga

There are many different styles of yoga being taught and practiced today. All types of yoga are based on the same physical postures, called "asanas", and each different posture helps the body in a unique way. Below is a quick guide to the most popular types of yoga. You might want to try a few different yoga classes to figure out what type is right for you.

Hatha Yoga

Hatha is a very general term that can include many types of yoga combined. If a class is described as Hatha style, it is probably going to be slow-paced and gentle and can provide a good introduction to basic yoga poses.

Vinyasa Yoga

Like Hatha, Vinyasa is a general term used to describe many different types of yoga combined. As Vinyasa means "breath-synchronized movement," it tends to be a more vigorous style of yoga based on a series of poses called "sun salutations" where your movements are matched to your breath. Towards the end of a Vinyasa class, there is also intense stretching.

Ashtanga and Power Yoga

Ashtanga, which means "eight limbs" in Sanskrit, is a fast-paced, intense style of yoga. With this yoga, a regular series of poses is generally performed in the same order and ideally in a heated room to simulate the warm temperature in India where yoga originated. Ashtanga yoga is physically demanding due to the constant flow from one pose to the next. This type of yoga has also been the inspiration for Power Yoga, based on a flowing style but without the strict set of regular poses. Be prepared to sweat in these classes!

Iyengar Yoga

Based on the teachings of Yogi B.K.S Iyengar, this style of yoga is all about body alignment. In yoga, the word "alignment" is used to describe the precise way your body should be positioned in each pose in order to obtain the maximum benefits and to avoid injury. Iyengar yoga usually emphasizes holding poses over long periods of time versus moving quickly from one pose to another. This type of yoga also incorporates the use of props such as yoga blankets, blocks and straps to bring the body into alignment.

Kundalini Yoga

The emphasis in Kundalini yoga is on the breath in conjunction with physical movement. The intention of this kind of yoga is to free the energy in your lower body and allow it to move upwards toward your upper glands and chakras (energy centers). Kundalini may include rapid, repetitive movements rather than static poses. There are thousands of kriyas (yoga sets of poses) in Kundalini yoga and meditation is always an integral component of it. Some kriyas and meditations may also involve the use of sounds or mantras.

Bikram or Hot Yoga

Pioneered by Bikram Choudhury, Bikram yoga is practiced in a 95 -100 degree (Fahrenheit) room; the principle is that the heat helps loosen tight muscles and cleanse the body through profuse sweating. In Bikram yoga, much like Ashtanga yoga, a regular series of poses is performed in the same order and is generally repeated once. It can take time to become acclimatized to the heat of the room.

Anusara Yoga

Founded in 1997 by John Friend, Anusara yoga focuses on physical alignment and a philosophy derived from Tantra which believes in the intrinsic goodness of all beings. Anusara classes are usually light-hearted and accessible to those of varying abilities. Poses are taught in a way that opens the heart physically and emotionally. Props are often used.

Jivamukti Yoga

This style of yoga emerged from teachers at a well-known New York yoga studio. Inspired by Ashtanga yoga, but wanting something a little different, Jivamukti yoga founders, David Life and Sharon Gannon, created a yoga that emphasized chanting, meditation and spiritual teachings along with movements from Ashtanga yoga.

Whatever type of yoga you choose to do, notice how it works your body, mind and soul. When you do start a yoga practice, go at your own pace; yoga is not a competitive sport!

ASK YOURSELF...

- What could yoga do for me?

- What type of yoga would be best for me?

- What type of exercise would benefit me the most at this time in my life?

YOUR WELLNESS STRATEGIES

- This week, look for a yoga class near you; perhaps in a yoga center or at your local gym.

- This week, attend a yoga class.

- This week, meditate for five to 10 minutes each day..

Note: Before you attempt any exercise program, please check with your doctor.

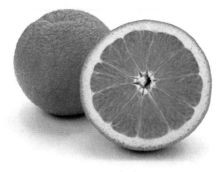

Chapter 25: Boning Up

– Dr. Nathalie

"Better to understand a little, than to misunderstand a lot."
– Anonymous

Cardiovascular exercise and muscle strength are important, but let's not forget the importance of strong bones. Did you know that there are 208 bones in the human body and 143 joints? Think how smart you'll look when you mention that around the water cooler at work tomorrow. If any of these joints or bones weaken, it can throw your body mechanics out of balance, affecting your overall physical health. And wouldn't you rather stand straight in your old age than hunched over, likely in some degree of chronic pain? Each year about 2.5 million North American men and women suffer a broken bone as a result of bone strength deterioration.

Osteoarthritis

Osteoarthritis is derived from the Greek word *osteo*, meaning 'of the bone'; *arthro*, meaning 'joint'; and *itis*, meaning 'inflammation'. Osteoarthritis is a condition in which low-grade inflammation results in pain in the joints caused by the wear and tear of the cartilage that covers and cushions the joints. Osteoarthritis is the most common form of arthritis.

I like to simplify things with my patients by telling them that osteoarthritis is the wear and tear on their spine and joints caused, in most cases, by overuse or improper joint mechanics. Like a car part that's not installed correctly, the spine will wear out much faster. It's the same thing with our joints. Unlike a car, though, we can't replace our parts!! So, it's all about prevention, maintaining and achieving optimal function of the spine and joints.

Osteoporosis

Osteoporosis is also derived from the Greek translation of the word *osteo*, meaning bones; *poro*, meaning 'porous'; and *osis,* meaning 'condition of'. Osteoporosis is a generalized disorder of skeletal bones in which the quantity and the quality of the bone tissue is decreased and the bone becomes weak and susceptible to breaking. 'Osteopenia' is a condition that occurs before osteoporosis and signifies that you've had *some* bone density and strength loss. This is a warning sign that osteoporosis is on the horizon. Proper nutrition, supplementation and exercise starting in childhood are imperative for proper bone growth, but it's never too late to make a difference in your bone health.

Osteoporosis is particularly problematic for women once they start menopause. Post-menopausal women have reduced levels of the hormone estrogen, which accelerates the leaching of calcium from bones. Hormone replacement therapy, which was popular until a few years ago, was shown to indeed reduce bone loss but, unfortunately, it also increased the risks of breast cancer, blood clots, heart attack and stroke.

In the case of osteoporosis, we're talking about the density of your bones. As an example, I tell my patients to think about putting a healthy bone and an osteoporotic bone in a tank of water. The healthy bone would sink to the bottom because it's dense while the osteoporotic bone would float because it's less dense (more porous).

Bone Density Measurement

Different tools are used to measure osteoarthritis and osteoporosis. Unfortunately both conditions can be present at the same time. Osteoarthritis can be seen on plain film X-rays, with a CT scan, or an MRI. Osteoporosis, however, needs to be measured by a Bone Mineral Density (BMD) test. There are a variety of these tests that do everything from measuring your hip, spine, wrist, finger, shin bone and heel to determine bone mass. These tests will measure your bone mineral density against that of a healthy 30-year-old and you will then be provided with a 'T-score'.

Results

- A T-Score of -1.0 and above indicates normal bone density;

- A T-score of -1.0 to -2.5 indicates that a person is considered to have low bone mass – osteopenia;

- A score below -2.5 indicates osteoporosis.

There is some controversy over the interpretation of the significance of these readings. Some experts believe that Bone Densitometry Testing predicts the risk of fracture in much the same way that a cholesterol reading is said to predict the risk of heart disease and blood pressure tests are said to predict the risk of stroke. Others say that bone density is more like a measure of a condition, not necessarily a disease in and of itself.

So, how did osteoporosis go from being considered a rare but serious disease to an epidemic that strikes fear in middle-aged women across North America? One answer may be the degree to which pharmaceutical companies market and promote their products to induce fear of developing osteoporosis. There has been a large increase in the number of bone-measuring devices and an increase in awareness campaigns to medical practitioners and patients about osteoporosis. While that may seem like a positive step, it's important to understand that the motivation behind such campaigns may be, in part, to sell more drugs.

Several drugs are approved for the prevention and treatment of osteoporosis (biphosphonates) and do indeed help with bone loss, but none are 100 percent effective, and, like all drugs, they come with side effects such as upper gastrointestinal pain and erosion, esophagitis, ulcers, skin rash, diffuse bone pain, and osteonecrosis (bone death) of the jaw. Another fact to take into consideration is that bones are dynamic structures and consistently need a balance between the bone-forming cells (osteoblasts) and the bone-destroying cells (osteoclasts) to keep them strong.

Some biphosphonate drugs used to treat osteoporosis stop and kill osteoclasts, thereby decreasing the bone destruction rate, but these drugs do not help promote osteoblasts (responsible for bone growth); they actually decrease their activity. In other words, the biphosphonate drugs may slow down deterioration, but they don't necessarily help the existing damage nor new bone formation. It's even been suggested that their anti-bone remodeling action may actually make bones more brittle and more prone to fracture over time.

Another strike against biphosphonate drugs is that they also decrease available calcium in your blood, which would have been obtained by normal osteoclasts activity. Calcium is an important buffer in the body and decreasing its access can play a major role in creating an acidity/alkalinity imbalance. As discussed in previous chapters, an acidic body will set the stage for disease. Biphosphonate drugs have also been shown to stay in the body for years.

Before starting on potentially dangerous drug therapy at the first sign of bone loss, educate yourself on the role of nutrition and exercise to ensure optimal bone health. That is why, when possible, prevention should be started at a young age!

Calcium – Its Other Role

Calcium is the most common mineral in your body. Your bones have very high calcium content but calcium is also essential to many physiological functions and if you don't have enough of it, your body will take what it needs from your bones to maintain adequate calcium levels. Your body needs calcium for functions like clotting, regulating heart beat, conducting nerve impulses, stimulating hormone secretions and muscle contractions.

As mentioned previously, calcium also has an important role as a buffer. For example, if you consume a soft drink, your body may have to take calcium from your bones to buffer the acidity of the beverage. Research shows that the average diet of a North American is very acidic, which can cause a myriad of health problems if left unchecked (see chapter #17 – "Adjusting Your Inner PH For Optimal Health"). Soft drinks are high in phosphoric acid and sugar, making them very acidic. The phosphoric acid necessitates calcium and potassium to neutralize the acidity. It does that by leaching calcium from our bones. When it comes to our children, one third of all drinks consumed by adolescents are soft drinks. Is it any wonder that bone-building is being compromised during peak growth years? Note that a diet high in sugar has also been shown to upset calcium and phosphorous balance in the body.

Milk – Maybe Not so Good!

It's commonly thought that dairy products are good sources of calcium; however, they may not be the best source. Cow's milk is rich in phosphorous, and when combined with calcium can actually prevent it from being absorbed properly. The protein in milk may also cause calcium to leach out of the bones. When you consider that many dairy cows may have been injected with antibiotics, leading to antibiotic resistance, it may not be the best calcium source for our families. Bovine growth hormones, while illegal in Canada, are still used in some countries to yield more milk per cow. Another factor to consider is that many people are sensitive to cow's milk, not just to the lactose in the milk but the protein in milk itself, which may lead, for example, to gastro-intestinal problems, allergies and eczema.

In some aspects, organic milk is a better alternative than regular milk, but there is a concern over the pasteurization process. When milk is pasteurized all the important enzymes are destroyed and, without these enzymes, milk becomes difficult to digest, placing added stress on the pancreas, which may lead to diabetes.

Other Sources of Calcium

Besides dairy, other sources of calcium include:

- Broccoli
- Collards
- Kale
- Mustard greens
- Turnip greens
- Bok choy or Chinese cabbage
- Salmon
- Sardines canned with their soft bones
- Shellfish
- Almonds
- Brazil nuts
- Dried beans

The Best Calcium Supplement

As for the best form of calcium to take, there are a lot of opinions and products out there. According to the book, The Bone Building Solution, by Dr. Graci, Dr. Demarco and Dr. Rao, the most clinically proven, soluble and absorbable forms of calcium for human consumption are: calcium bisglycinate, calcium formate and calcium citrate-malate.

Other recommendations include a blend of different ingredients – citrate, gluconate, carbonate, lactate, ascorbate, malate and micro-crystalline hydroxyapatite. Keep in mind that everyone metabolizes supplements a little differently and that different sources of calcium are also absorbed differently. A broad spectrum calcium supplement, however, will work for a broad spectrum of people. For instance, calcium carbonate is only 40 percent calcium by weight, so a 500 mg tablet will only contain 200 mg of actual calcium. Calcium citrate only contains 21 percent calcium by weight, so a 500 mg tablet only has 105 mg of calcium. Despite the fact it has a lower calcium component than calcium carbonate; calcium citrate is absorbed better by the body than calcium carbonate.

When taking a calcium supplement, most experts agree that no more than 500 mg of calcium should be taken at one time. The percentage of calcium absorbed decreases as the amount of calcium in the supplement increases. The body needs approximately 1,000 to 1,500 mg of calcium per day. Spreading your doses throughout the day will increase absorption. It may be beneficial to take your calcium supplement in the evening as it has a relaxing effect on the muscles and could even help you sleep better!

Calcium Absorption

For calcium to be absorbed and utilized adequately by your body it needs help – this is why you will rarely see calcium supplements sold on their own. For optimal absorption, calcium needs to be taken in conjunction with:

- Magnesium
- Vitamin C
- Vitamin D

The best source of vitamin D is the sun. Depending on how much you already have in your diet and whether you are routinely exposed to a lot of sunlight, daily recommended intake is between 800IU and 1000IU. Most North Americans are deficient in vitamin D and new research shows an important correlation between several cancers and vitamin D deficiency, as well as other major health issues (see chapter #26 – "Vitamin D, Sunshine And Sunscreen").

The absorption of calcium also depends on the level of acidity in the stomach – insufficient levels of hydrochloric acid (HCL) decreases calcium absorption which can lead to osteoporosis. So be aware that digestive aids promoting their calcium content, not only decrease the amount of gastric acid in your stomach but may make the body unable to absorb the calcium in the tablets.

Since calcium is absorbed mostly in the bowel, it's important to have efficient bowel function for optimal absorption. The intestine has good bacteria to digest and breakdown our food, but it also has bad bacteria known as Candida Albicans. Good bacteria in the bowels should not be out-numbered by bad bacteria. A sign of increasing bad bacteria in your bowel is bloating and gas after eating. The use of good probiotics will help you with good bowel health, thereby creating optimal nutrient absorption.

Other Elements Required for Bone Health:

- Protein for the basic framework of the bone
- Copper, zinc, manganese, silica and boron, selenium – important co-factors for aiding calcium absorption
- Vitamin K1, K2 and the presence of "good" intestinal bacteria
- Lycopene, which helps bones stay strong and disease-free
- Fish oil – EPA and DHA – increases calcium absorption and reduces inflammation
- Weight-bearing exercises that put stress on your bones which makes them react and grow stronger
- An alkaline body – acidity promotes bone loss
- Avoid sodas as they too, promote bone loss

New, promising, quality natural products like OsteoDenx™ from Nikken are designed to promote both aspects of bone health. These aspects are the release/absorption of vital mineral compounds and the formation of new bone tissue. This product is not a calcium supplement or a medication. It features a patented Syno-portin™ technology that enables vital bone health ingredients to reach the specific target sites of absorption. This offers increased bioavailability, so that more of these ingredients will be assimilated by bone tissue.

Promoting optimal balance of these materials within bones and joints helps maintain bone density and supports the structure and integrity of cartilage. Recent research results conclude that ribonuclease-enriched lactoferrin supplementation (which is a component of OsteoDenx™) demonstrates a statistically significant reduction in bone resorption and an increase in osteoblastic bone formation. This proves to help restore the balance of bone turnover within a short period of time.

Again, remember the importance of weight bearing exercise to put "stress" on your bones and make them stronger!

In a nutshell, if you wish to decrease your chances of developing osteoporosis:

- Eat more fruits and vegetables
- Maintain a consistent exercise program including weight bearing exercises (yes ladies – lift those weights!)
- Avoid soft drinks
- Avoid smoking, excess alcohol and sugar
- Increase your intake of alkaline food and decrease your intake of acidic food
- Take a good quality multivitamin
- Supplement your diet with adequate calcium, magnesium, vitamin D and vitamin C
- Supplement with other bone-supporting elements, such as OsteoDenx™, to increase the delivery of calcium to the bone

ASK YOURSELF...

- Is my current diet rich in bone-building nutrients?
- Do I engage in daily weight-bearing exercises?
- Do I need to complement my diet with bone-building supplements?

YOUR WELLNESS STRATEGIES

- List three actions you can start doing today to ensure better bone health (e.g. increase calcium-rich foods in your diet, take supplements, get more sun for vitamin D and start a weight training program). If you consume soft drinks, try substituting water at least once a day. Encourage your children to do the same.

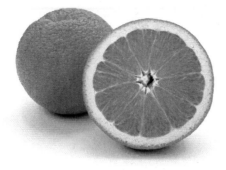

Chapter 26: Vitamin D, Sunshine And Sunscreen

– Dr. Nathalie

"If you believe everything you read, you better not read."
– Japanese Proverb

Sunshine is a vital ingredient for staying healthy and is your best source for essential vitamin D. Sunlight also provides you with numerous other health benefits such as fighting depression. In recent studies, vitamin D has been shown to even protect against several types of cancer. As discussed in our chapter on bone health, vitamin D is also important for proper absorption of calcium and in maintaining strong bones.

We hear a lot about skin cancer due to overexposure to the sun, but did you know that tens of thousands of North Americans die of cancer and other illnesses every year due to inadequate sun exposure and dire levels of vitamin D? In the U.S., the annual cost of treating illnesses due to the lack of sun exposure hovers around $56 billion – and only $6 billion is spent on treating illnesses due to overexposure to sunlight. Of course, it's true that the sun can cause cancer when skin is exposed to excess amounts, so it's important to avoid getting sunburned. But don't avoid the sun altogether as it is still the best source of vitamin D and is better than taking it in tablets!

Understanding Ultraviolet

Most people are aware of the effects of Ultra Violet (UV) rays through painful sunburns, but the UV spectrum has many other effects, both beneficial and detrimental to our health. Darker-skinned people, however, will produce more of the natural skin-protecting substance called 'eumelanin', which may offer some protection from the negative effects of UVB and UVA.

For starters, it's important to be UV-knowledgeable; the sun emits ultraviolet radiation in UVA, UVB, and UVC rays and not all rays are created equal.

UVC: UVC rays are filtered out by the stratosphere so they are of little concern.

UVB: UVB rays are responsible for vitamin D production – something your body benefits from. On the downside, UVB rays are also responsible for sunburn and damage to the surface of the skin. These rays cause moles, skin aging and some types of skin cancer. UVB rays only make up a fraction of UV light.

UVA: Looking at UVA in a "positive light", these will not cause sunburn but rather a tan and they cause less cancer than UVB rays. UVA rays make up the majority of UV light.

Unfortunately, the cancer that UVA rays do cause is the most dangerous – melanoma. It also contributes more to skin aging and DNA damage than UVB ray and often times is less effectively blocked by sunscreens.

Skin Cancer

Skin cancer represents the most commonly diagnosed malignancy, surpassing lung, breast, colorectal and prostate cancer. But despite what we have been led to believe, a reasonable amount of sun exposure reduces the risk of skin cancer because of the vitamin D stimulated by skin exposure to sunlight.

Another point to take into consideration is that skin cancers have been linked to a large disproportion in the ratio of Omega-6 to Omega-3. Our North American diets are often much higher in Omega-6 and may place us at a greater risk of developing skin cancer. Increasing your intake of Omega-3 is therefore very important to rebalance your Omega-6 to Omega-3 ratio.

The three main types of skin cancer are: 1) Basal Cell Carcinoma; 2) Squamous Cell Carcinoma and 3) Malignant Melanoma. The first two are the most common types of cancer but are mostly localized and are more easily treated. Melanoma, however, while rare, is potentially fatal.

Sunscreen

How do sunscreens work? Chemical agents in sunscreens absorb the sun's UV rays and convert them into harmless thermal energy or reflect it off the body. While this product may help protect from sunburns, you need to be aware of the chemicals in your sunscreen and whether they might pose more of a health risk than the sun itself. Sunscreen may protect from the sun, but if you think the lotion is harmless, think again...Your skin is the largest organ in your body and everything that you put on it is absorbed into your blood stream. Just think about nicotine or estrogen patches and how they work. So, as a rule, knowing that everything that goes on you, ends up in you, you shouldn't put anything on your skin that you wouldn't ingest. Now go read the ingredient list on a bottle of sunscreen; would you willingly eat any of that?

Studies have shown that those who use sunscreen actually have a higher risk of skin cancer than those who don't. One study reported that the greatest increase in melanoma occurred in regions where sunscreen use is most prevalent and another one showed a higher incidence of basal cell carcinoma in women who used sunscreens. In fact sunscreen is linked to about 150,000 cancer cases every year. They have also been shown to:

- Act like estrogen and disrupt hormones
- Cause allergic reactions
- Accumulate in the body

Sunscreen can actually block the absorption of vitamin D, and studies have shown that vitamin D can prevent up to 77 types of cancers.

So all that said, sunscreens are effective in reducing sunburns, but may not reduce the risk of cancer. The debate over sunscreen, however, is still ongoing and while the debate ensues, you need to educate yourself about sunscreen. The first question that needs to be answered concerns SPF – what is it?

SPF is actually a test designed to measure how much a product protects against UVB rays. It does not test the protection against UVA rays. For this reason, it gives many a false sense of protection against the sun and many may stay out longer because of it.

There are, however, products on the market that provide protection against both UVA and UVB rays; they contain ingredients like zinc oxide and titanium dioxide, and they won't break down in the sun's extreme heat like other ingredients could. Unfortunately, regulatory bodies have not yet fully established proper standards for the efficacy or the safety of sunscreen ingredients. In fact, sunscreen manufacturers are free to market products that haven't been proven to protect from the sun.

At the time of writing, The Environmental Working Group has assessed over 830 sunscreens on the market and uncovered that only 16 percent actually provide adequate protection from both UVA and UVB radiation without the added toxins. Visit www.cosmeticsdatabase.com to find out more.

Finding a natural, non-toxic, full-spectrum sunscreen is the way to go. Ultimately, the ideal sunscreen is both kid- and adult-friendly, highly effective at blocking UVA and UVB rays, and doesn't have ingredients that break down in the sun. Make sure also you don't combine it with bug repellent, because the ingredients in the repellent will make you absorb a higher amount of the chemicals present. Remember that everything you put on your skin is absorbed by your body. So, be aware of that fact when buying repellent. What are you spraying on your children? Yet another example of the power of marketing!

One other option to protect yourself from the sun – if you have to be outside for a while, is to buy some UV- resistant clothing – they come with protective factors as high as 40.

Tanning Beds and Creams

For some people, getting vitamin D from the sun is not easy, especially during the winter months. It is possible to get a vitamin D boost from a tanning bed or booth but UV radiation in tanning beds can be as much as 15 times higher than the sun's. Some experts suggest asking for a tanning bed with a high UVB to UVA ratio – since only UVB produces vitamin D.

Also, the electromagnetic fields (EMF) emitted by the magnetic ballasts in tanning beds are of concern. Newer beds tend to have lower EMFs and tend to use more electronic ballast types which will help make them safer. You will need to research each tanning salon individually to find out more about the safety of the beds they are using. And before you turn to self-tanning creams, be aware that they have not been tested for safety and contain multiple chemicals which can be toxic to your body. Don't be seduced by the nice self-tanning, cool-looking bottles; remember that everything you put on your skin is absorbed right into your blood stream!

Other Tips to Protect Yourself

- Avoid being in the sun from 10:00 a.m. to 2:00 p.m.;

- Cover yourself with light clothing if you're going to be out; gauge whether you need to do this based on how fair you are and how much you're exposed to sunlight on a regular basis;

- When spring/summer arrives, expose yourself gradually to the sun and let your skin adapt;

- Make sure you wear sunglasses that protect your eyes from UVA and UVB rays.

ASK YOURSELF...

- Do I spend at least 15 minutes (longer if you have naturally darker skin) in the sun every day to get my minimum recommended intake of daily vitamin D (800IU to 1000IU)?

- Do I overexpose myself to the sun and get sunburned regularly?

- What chemicals does my sunscreen contain?

- Have I looked for a more "natural" sunscreen at my local health food store?

YOUR WELLNESS STRATEGIES

- Go outside for at least 15 minutes every day, starting today.

- If you're going to be outside for a long period of time protect yourself with clothing, sunscreen, or stay in the shade.

- Buy a more "natural" sunscreen to protect yourself and your family.

- If you use a tanning bed, inquire about its EMFs, UVB to UVA ratio and the different types of ballasts used.

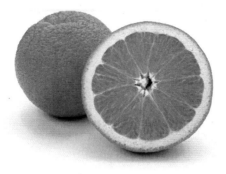

Chapter 27: Laughter Is The Sunshine Of Your Life

– Andrée

"The art of medicine consists of keeping the patient amused while nature heals the disease."

– Voltaire

Children know how to laugh; watch them at play and count how many times they laugh in 30 minutes. Notice how spontaneous it is. They smile at things that adults might consider silly but it's genuine happiness. Children laugh up to 300 times each day in comparison with adults who laugh 17 times each day. While some adults have made the conscious decision not to laugh as much – perhaps because they think it's childish – others have simply forgotten because the pressures and stresses of life have taken over.

We're going to jump-start your laughter sensors again and here's why…

Do you remember the scene in the movie Mary Poppins, when Uncle Albert, an older gentleman, starts laughing uncontrollably and as he does he levitates to the ceiling? Proving that laughter is contagious, actor Dick Van Dyke, "Bert" in the movie, begins laughing as well and he too levitates, as do the children. The more they laughed the higher they went – a drug-free high! This is a beautiful representation of what laughter can do – it can lighten and lift us up! Think about it, laughing makes you feel lighter, brighter and full of life. Who doesn't want more of that?

Benefits of Laughter

There are other reasons why laughter is good for you too. Health-wise, laughter generates endorphins in your body, natural feel-good chemicals. This natural high can last for up to 12 hours – talk about a good day.

Studies have shown that people who laugh on a regular basis have lower blood pressure. When you laugh, your blood pressure first increases but then decreases lower than it was before. Your breathing also becomes deeper, giving your body more oxygen.

If you want to keep your heart healthy, laughter is the best medicine for that too. A study from the University of Maryland showed that laughing helps prevent heart disease. The study found that people with heart disease were 40 percent less likely to laugh than others.

Laughter also gives your body an awesome workout. It works your diaphragm, abdominal muscles, lungs, facial muscles, legs, and even buttock muscles! It can help with digestion and food absorption…in fact, a good laugh can burn as many calories as a rowing machine in the same amount of time.

In addition, laughter is a powerful emotional medicine that can lower your stress level in the blink of an eye. Laughing in a tense situation will help relax your muscles and prevent psychological strain. How you react to events and situations is what causes the stress. Mental health professionals have noted how humor can shift the way you think. It's important to have a healthy sense of humor that includes being able to laugh at yourself and events in your life. Laugh at yourself when it's called for and realize that not every dilemma is earth-shattering; some situations are quite insignificant and don't need to be taken so seriously. Laughter and humor can adjust the meaning of an event so that it's not so overwhelming. When you do this you accept and respect who you are and where you are in your life.

Why Laughter is Essential

The mental health benefits of laughter…

- Enhances your ability to connect with others
- Encourages you to talk more, make more eye and body contact with others
- Replaces distressing emotions with pleasurable feelings

The physical health benefits of laughter…

- Increases energy
- Reduces stress
- Lowers blood pressure
- Boosts immune system
- Protects the heart
- Improves brain function
- Promotes attentiveness
- Exercises the facial muscles – maybe prevent a wrinkle or two!
- Fosters relaxation

So go on, be a kid again, laugh! You look funny trying to be so serious!

Laughter Yoga

For those of you who have trouble laughing naturally, there's a fabulous exercise called Laughter Yoga. First developed in India, Laughter Yoga is now practiced in 53 countries around the world.

In Laughter Yoga, you pretend to find things funny, forcing the laughter. The beauty of it is, it has the same effect on the body as natural laughter. Miraculously, after attending one of these classes you'll actually feel happier. With each Laughter Yoga class, laughter will come easier to you. Plus you'll be more relaxed and you may even see sleep improvements.

ASK YOURSELF…

- How many times each day do I think I laugh?
- Can I easily laugh at myself, without putting myself down?
- When was the last time I had a good belly laugh?

Your Wellness Strategies

- Look for situations or events this week that you can laugh at instead of dramatizing them.

- Watch a comedy film this weekend and give yourself permission to laugh out loud.

- Visualize a past event that made you laugh uncontrollably and laugh at it again.

- See if a Laughter Yoga class is being offered near you and give it a try.

- Pick up Loretta Laroche's CD, "Life is Short, Wear Your Party Pants!" – I dare you not to laugh!

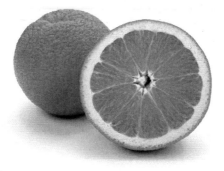

Chapter 28: "Whey" To Go!

– Dr. Nathalie

"Strong reasons make strong actions."
– William Shakespeare

Should you supplement your diet with whey protein? "I don't work out," you might think, or "Taking more protein will make me get big, bulky or fat." Believe it or not, these are the comments I get from my female patients when I suggest they take a whey supplement. First of all, let's get something straight – you won't look bulky by taking protein supplements! I have news for you ladies – you need protein too! Read on…

Whey protein is a simple and convenient way to boost your protein intake (and can complement a whole-food diet) – especially on-the-go for all of us with busy lifestyles. Whey comes in powder form, easy to spoon into a shaker and then just add water whenever and wherever you're ready for it. Et voilà!

Whey is actually a by-product of cow's milk. It's not a new phenomenon but has gained popularity in the last couple of decades in the sports nutrition industry for giving athletes the nutrition they need to be their best.

What is whey? A high quality protein source, whey is a co-product of the cheese-making process, derived from milk solids. The composition of whole milk includes: 87 percent water and 13 percent milk solids. From that 13 percent of milk solids come: 30 percent fat, 37 percent lactose, <u>27 percent protein</u>, and six percent ash and minerals. From that 27 percent protein comes <u>20 percent whey protein</u> and 80 percent casein. A long process to get there, but well worth it for us.

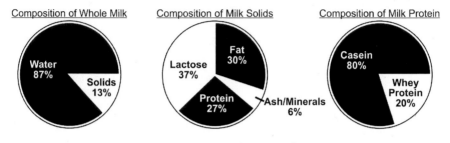

Composition of Whole Milk   Composition of Milk Solids   Composition of Milk Protein

Whey protein has a mixture of proteins with different biological properties. These proteins are: beta-lactoglobulin, alpha-lactoalbumin, bovine serum albumin, immunoglobulin, and lactoferrin to name a few.

Benefits of Whey Protein

Whey is a high-quality protein complete with all the essential amino acids your body must acquire through diet. While your body is able to make non-essential amino acids from other amino acids in your system, it can't make essential amino acids like the ones that come from whey. The only solution is to include essential amino acids by ingesting them in high-quality protein foods. Protein sources that contain all of the essential amino acids are called complete proteins; whey is one of these. Essential amino acids are the building blocks for healthy muscles, skin, nails and other body tissues.

Studies show that whey protein may:

- Potentially reduce cancer
- Help fight HIV
- Improve immunity
- Reduce stress
- Lower cholesterol
- Improve liver function
- Reduce blood pressure
- Improve athletic performance

- Improve blood sugar regulation – another key to controlling appetite and metabolism

Whey protein also has an effect on certain hormones in the body, like cholecystokinin, a hormone responsible for the feeling of satiety after a meal. Feeling fuller for longer could decrease your overall food intake.

The tryptophan in whey will also play a role in increasing your body's serotonin hormone levels. Serotonin is linked to mood, anxiety levels and appetite. An increase in serotonin will make you feel happy, relaxed and full.

Whey also boosts glutathione concentration. Glutathione is an important component of your body's antioxidant defense system and protects your cells against free radical damage, pollution, toxins and infection. Glutathione levels decrease with age and this decline is associated with the onset of many age-related diseases.

Recent studies show that consuming whey protein and doing resistance training exercises will help you build valuable muscle mass and maintain that mass as you age. Whey shows the best results compared to any other supplement when it comes to achieving a lean body composition.

Different Types of Whey

1. *Whey concentrate*

   Years ago, whey only contained 30 percent to 40 percent of protein and high amounts of lactose and fat. Now, due to better procedure, whey concentrate can have as much as 70 percent to 80 percent protein and reduced lactose and fat.

2. *Whey isolates*

   Whey protein isolate will contain as much as 90 percent to 96 percent of protein, minimal lactose and virtually no fat. In order to keep the protein quality this high, the whey must be processed under low temperatures and with low acid conditions so as not to denature (breakdown) the protein.

   - *Whey isolate – Ion exchange*

     While whey produced through ion exchange is high in protein, it is a procedure with serious drawbacks as it uses chemicals like hydrochloric acid and sodium hydroxide during processing.

Because of this, the most important components of the whey, sub-fraction peptides which boost health and immunity, are depleted.

- *Whey isolate – Micro-filtered*

Micro-filtered whey isolate is very high in protein while retaining the important sub-fraction peptides. Proteins are also not denatured. It is also extremely low in fat and lactose.

Narrow Your Whey Search

- Look for a whey product that does not have artificial sweeteners like Aspartame®, Succaryl ®, or Splenda ® in it. Keep in mind that artificial sweeteners are toxic to the body and linked to obesity and several chronic illnesses. Sweet alternatives found in nature are stevia, which come in liquid or powder form or Lu-Hon which is a fruit extract. Another choice is agave nectar which has a beneficial Low Glycemic Index. If you must use an artificial sweetener, Xylitol is a less harmful option. But Xylitol is a sugar alcohol and could lead to gastro-intestinal discomfort if used in big quantities.

- Because whey protein comes from cows, it is best to find a product that states the cows are grass fed, free of pesticides, and not given hormones or antibiotics. Organic whey protein may be difficult to find as it's limited in its supply – but is best in a perfect world.

- Try buying micro-filtered whey isolate as it has the highest protein content and will also give your body the best health and immune benefits.

Whey Protein and Meal Replacement

There is a difference between protein supplements and meal replacements. A protein supplement will have mostly protein in it and very little carbs or fat. A meal replacement will, however, contain protein, carbs and fat. Depending on what kind of supplementation you actually need, both can be beneficial. But be aware that by consuming a meal replacement you're increasing your caloric intake, so unless you're trying to gain weight, you need to be careful. It is a good alternative for example, if you need to miss a meal for a practical reason but don't want to skimp on nutrition. Again, be aware of the type of sweetener used in the meal replacement you buy.

Other Additions to Whey Protein Supplements

Often times you will see a lot of additives in whey protein supplements – vitamins, glutamine, conjugated Linoleic Acid, etc. Depending on your specific needs you may not require all those extras, especially if you have a well-balanced, whole food diet and you're taking a good multivitamin (see chapter #11 – "Do We Need Multivitamins? Are They All Created Equal?"). If you are not getting the proper nutrients from your diet, if you are an athlete putting a lot of stress on your body by exercising very frequently, or if you are just under a lot of stress, you may, however, benefit from those additions.

How Much To Use

Typically, a serving of 20 to 40 grams of whey protein is suggested. You can take whey before or after your workout. What you eat before a workout – carbs, fats and proteins – dictates what you'll burn for energy. Research suggests that taking whey before exercise can help you burn more fat and build more muscle. Taking whey after exercise is also very beneficial as it is rapidly digested and absorbed by your body, providing a supply of amino acids/protein to your muscles for repair and recovery.

If you are by chance lactose-intolerant, you should use a pure whey protein *isolate* as it has less then 0.1 grams of lactose per tablespoon. Protein *concentrate* should be avoided by the lactose-intolerant as it usually contains a fair amount of lactose.

ASK YOURSELF...

- When my energy is low, do I reach for that high-carb, no-nutrient snack?

- Is my daily protein intake adequate? (See chapter # 5 – "Protein, Carbs And Fat – What Am I Eating?").

- Am I often sick – could I use whey protein to improve my immune system?

- Do I know which type/brand of protein to use?

- If I am already using whey protein, have I read the labels to see what artificial sweeteners are used, if any?

YOUR WELLNESS STRATEGIES

- Talk to someone at your local health food store or to your natural health care provider, and find out what choices are available near you.

- Find a brand of whey protein that does not have artificial sweetener in it.

- Prepare your whey protein ahead of time so that you just have to add water when you need it on-the-go.

- Add a scoop of whey protein to your green drink for a great power drink!

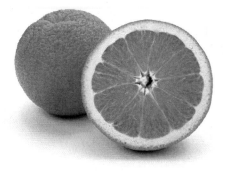

Chapter 29: The Soy Controversy

– Dr. Nathalie

*"All truths are easy to understand once they are discovered;
the point is to discover them."*

– Galileo Galilei

More shocking information! Up until not too long ago, I too was drinking my soy milk and trying really hard to replace my cheese with soy cheese. Little did I know that I had fallen prey to a multi-billion dollar marketing machine that was trying to convince me to buy something that I later found out may not be so great for me. It was only when I started doing my own research on soy products that I discovered the real story behind this so-called health wonder.

Depending on your sources, you can probably find as many good reasons to consume soy products as reasons to avoid them! One thing I will ask you to consider is the source of the information and who benefits from it. Money talks (the soy industry is a multi-billion dollar industry), so we have to consider that all organizations and administrations do not necessarily have our well-being at the top of their priority list and that research can, at times, be self-serving. The book, The Whole Soy Story, by Dr. Kaayla T. Daniel, is a great resource book and was a big eye-opener for me.

My goal in writing this chapter was again to make you *aware* of the controversy on the subject by presenting you with the pros and cons of consuming soy. With this information at hand, I hope you will be able to make a more educated decision on *your* soy consumption.

The History of Soy

Until a few decades ago, with the discovery of fermentation techniques, the soybean was considered unfit to eat, even in Asia. Contrary to popular belief, Asian diets include only small amounts of soy, about nine grams per day, and not the processed kind of soy that North Americans eat. In contrast, in North America, one soy snack contains about 20 grams of non-fermented, processed soy. On top of being processed, a very large amount of soy crops are genetically modified and have been exposed to large amounts of herbicides and pesticides, leading to new compounds entering the body and causing associated concerns.

Today, every part of a soybean is used for profit. Soy protein isolate, which was initially invented to make cardboard, is now used in many of the food products we eat. And soy lecithin, also a regular ingredient, is actually the left-over waste of the soybean process.

Not-Soy-Good

Soybeans actually contain large quantities of natural toxins or "anti-nutrients" that inhibit good digestive enzymes. One of the inhibited enzymes is *trypsin*, needed for protein digestion. Without trypsin, you could develop serious gastric problems and chronic deficiencies related to amino acid uptake. Fermented soy products, however, decrease the amount of anti-nutrients present in the food and are thus easier to digest. The process of fermentation also destroys high amounts of phytates (on the outer layer of the bean) that can block the uptake of essential minerals – calcium, magnesium, copper, iron and zinc – in the intestinal tract. In addition, non-fermented soybeans contain *haemagglutinin*, which causes red blood cells to clump together and can significantly suppress growth. If you continue to consume soy products, choose those made from *fermented* beans. More on that later...

Other Effects of Soy

- There are studied risks of thyroid disturbances in those who consume soy – symptoms can be weight gain and lethargy;
- Soy can cause a bloated feeling after being consumed, also resulting in fatigue;

- According to Health Canada, soy is one of the nine most common food allergens;

- Soy can reduce fertility and libido in men; giving soy to monks to reduce libido is a well-known tradition in the East;

- Soy also may contain aluminum, which is a known neurotoxin to our bodies.

Soy Health Claims

1. *Soy and Heart Health*

- There are claims that soy decreases cholesterol levels.

- In 1999, the FDA authorized a health claim about the relationship between soy protein and Coronary Heart Disease (CHD) on the labelling of foods containing soy protein.

- Studies concerning the cholesterol-lowering effects of soy have been called immature. And while cholesterol-lowering products have fuelled a multi-billion dollar soy industry, heart disease has seen no decline.

2. *Soy, Menopause and Cancer*

- Soybeans contain the isoflavones genistein and daidzein. Those plant-based estrogens are called phytoestrogens or xeno-estrogen, meaning "foreign estrogen".

- Phytoestrogens can mimic human estrogen and bind to estrogen receptors in the human body. For this reason, researchers have proposed that soy phytoestrogen be used for natural hormone replacement therapy as the level of estrogen tends to drop after menopause, causing uncomfortable symptoms like hot flashes. However, even though isoflavones have been shown in some cases to have cancer-reducing effects, they have also been shown to promote hormone-sensitive cancers in some people. Studies are conflicting, because isoflavones affect people differently – even at extremely low levels.

- To be clear, while some studies suggest that soy protein may help prevent cancer, other studies show it is ineffective and inconsistent. Other studies reveal that soy phytoestrogen may actually increase the risk of developing breast cancer later on in life.

3. *Soy and Healthy Bones*

- Soy foods are naturally high in calcium which is great for bones. Unfortunately, soy is also high in phytic acid, which can block the uptake of essential minerals like calcium, magnesium, copper, iron and especially zinc.

- Soy protein can cause negative calcium balance and may even contribute to the development of osteoporosis.

- Vitamin K is also very important for bone health. Vitamin K2 is made in our body and produced by fermented food – so fermented soy can indeed be beneficial for bone density.

Soy Protein – Quality

Despite popular belief, soy has a low Biological Value score, which measures the actual amount of protein deposited per gram of protein absorbed. While whey receives a score of 104, whole eggs 100, and milk 94, soy receives a meager 74. The higher the BV, the better the protein.

Soybeans have been marketed as a complete protein but they are deficient in the amino acids (building blocks of proteins) methionine and cystine. Modern processing of the bean also may denature (break down) the amino acid lysine which will directly impact protein synthesis in our body.

Soy and Family Explained

- *Soybean oil* – soybeans are super heated, pressed, mixed with chemicals and washed in a centrifuge. In the U.S., soybean oil accounts for more than 75 percent of the total vegetable fats and oil intake – it's in all sorts of snack foods and fast foods. Soy bean oil is not fermented.

- *Soy milk* – a processed beverage made of ground soybeans mixed with water and boiled which actually removes some toxins. Soy milk is not fermented. Sugar is also added to improve flavor and an eight-ounce serving of this drink contains up to 35 milligrams of isoflavones, which may alter your estrogen levels and hinder hormone function. Since cow's milk has its own challenges – hormones, antibiotics, pesticides – it's a tough call. Organic milk is a better choice, but as mentioned previously, pasteurization destroys the good enzymes, reduces vitamin content and lowers the protein content. Another option is local, clean raw milk, rice milk (least allergenic), almond milk or water.

- *Tofu* – soy milk is curdled and pressed into cubes of varying firmness. Often used as a meat substitute, this product contains anti-nutrients (enzyme inhibitors). Contrary to popular belief, tofu is not fermented.

- *Edamame* – whole soybeans, commonly boiled in the pod and eaten as a snack. Most commercial edamame has been preheated to make digestion easier, but it still contains anti-nutrients.

- *Miso* – fermented soybean paste used in soups and sauces. This is rich in good bacteria that helps vitamin absorption. It's high in sodium, but it's considered one of the healthiest soy products around.

- *Tempeh* – whole soybeans are pressed into loaves and then fermented. Tempeh is rich in B vitamins, minerals and Omega-3 fatty acids.

- *Natto* – Soaked, boiled or steamed and then fermented, this whole-soybean product is a good source of vitamin K, which helps blood clotting and promotes healthy bones. Some, however, may not like the sticky texture and the rather foul smell!

Soy Baby Formula

Soy protein isolate is the main ingredient of soy-based infant formulas. Soy formulas are often given to babies with milk allergies, but allergies to soy are almost as common as those to milk. Infants fed soy formulas are exposed to high levels of isoflavones, which are potent anti-thyroid agents, and it may affect their normal growth and development. Soy formula will also adversely affect hormone levels by exposing infants to up to 2,000 times higher estrogen content. This increases the risk of behavioral problems. Soy formula also exposes infants to potentially high concentrations of aluminum and manganese. Soy formulas also lack cholesterol, which is absolutely essential for the development of the brain and nervous system.

Soy Protein Powder

Protein isolates from soy are also used in powder mixes intended for meal-replacement or protein drinks. These isolates are obtained by means of a high-temperature process that extensively denatures the protein. In its damaged form, the protein is rendered low in nutritional value. The soy protein isolates are also high in mineral-blocking phytates, thyroid-depressing phytoestrogen and potent enzyme inhibitors. As well, the high heat used in processing the isolates has been reported to increase the likelihood of forming carcinogenic compounds.

Final Soy Note

You may still want to use small amounts of organic *fermented* soy products in your diet; remember that fermented soy products like Miso, Tempeh and Natto can be beneficial for your health – it's all about balancing your diet and ensuring diversity in the foods you eat. Try to pass up non-fermented, processed soy products like milks, burgers, ice cream, and cheeses that are disguised as potential health foods. Also, be aware that most of what is labelled as "vegetable" oil is actually soybean oil so you may have a lot more soy hidden in your current diet than you think! (see chapter #5 – "Protein, Carbs, And Fat – What Am I Eating?").

ASK YOURSELF...

- How much soy do I consume on a daily basis?

- Have I ever looked at the ingredients of products I consume for their hidden soy content?

- Do I get bloated after consuming soy products?

- Do I experience intestinal problems and feel fatigue after eating soy products?

- Am I consuming the fermented or non-fermented soy products?

YOUR WELLNESS STRATEGIES

- Make a list of all the soy foods that you consume – fermented and non-fermented.

- Replace the non-fermented soy you eat with alternatives such as Miso, Tempeh and Natto.

- Find an alternative "milk" type (rice, almond or raw).

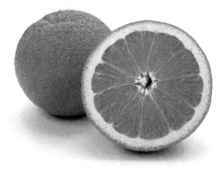

Chapter 30: Gluten – Are You Sensitive To it?

– Dr. Nathalie

"Nothing is as simple as we hope it will be."
– Jim Horning

Gluten is a protein found in all forms of wheat, rye, oats, barley and related hybrids. It is used in food processing because it binds, stabilizes and prevents crumbling. Celiac disease is a chronic intestinal mal-absorption disorder caused by intolerance to gluten. This hereditary disorder is caused by sensitivity to the gliadin fraction in gluten. When people who suffer from celiac disease consume gluten, the absorptive villi in the small intestine are damaged which prevents nutrients' absorption. Long-term effects, if untreated, can be very severe; but a gluten-free diet allows most patients to live a healthy and normal life.

Celiac experts estimated in a 2003 report that as many as one in every 133 Americans have the disease. Gluten sensitivity/intolerance on the other hand, is a condition that is easily under-diagnosed. It is often assumed to be a food allergy but is more an auto-immune process.

Some symptoms of gluten intolerance include:

- Recurring abdominal bloating and pain
- Chronic diarrhea
- Gas

- Bone pain
- Behavior changes
- Muscle cramps
- Fatigue and extreme weakness
- Pain of the joints
- Depression
- Seizures
- Tingling and numbness in the legs (from nerve damage)

Grains to avoid:

- Wheat – einkorn, emmer, spelt and kamut
- Wheat forms – wheat starch, wheat bran, wheat germ, cracked wheat, hydrolyzed wheat protein, farina, semolina, graham flour and durum flour
- Rye
- Barley
- Triticale (a cross between wheat and rye)

Grains allowed:

- Amaranth
- Buckwheat
- Corn
- Flax
- Millet
- Quinoa
- Rice
- Sorghum
- Wild Rice

Be aware that gluten is often hidden in things like soup, soy sauce or even candies. Make sure to read labels properly! Watch out for things like starch, malt, malt syrup, hydrolyzed vegetable protein (HVP) and texturized vegetable protein (TVP). You can get a more detailed list of foods that contain gluten and foods that are allowed while on a gluten-free diet in any good book on the topic or online.

The benefits of a gluten-free diet can be tremendous. People who suffer from gluten sensitivity will see improvements in the above mentioned symptoms within a short time and gluten can often be re-introduced in their diet when the irritation/inflammation of the bowel is gone. It can take up to one year for the bowel to completely heal. Studies show that people with rheumatoid arthritis, multiple sclerosis, Parkinson's disease, seizures, autism, ataxia (loss of balance), Down's syndrome, lymphoma, osteoporosis and diabetes may benefit considerably from living a gluten-free lifestyle.

ASK YOURSELF...

- Do I often feel bloated or in pain after a meal?

- Do I feel tired after eating?

- Do I often have gas, diarrhea or constipation?

- Is my diet high in gluten (e.g. wheat, rye and barley)?

YOUR WELLNESS STRATEGIES

- This week, try a gluten-free diet by avoiding the foods that contain gluten and notice how your digestive system feels. Notice your overall energy.

- Make a trip to the health food store and look at all the foods available that are gluten-free – educate yourself!

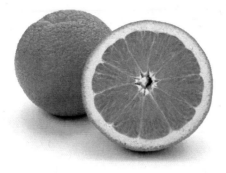

Chapter 31: Walking The Tightrope

– Andrée

"When awareness is completely balanced, communicating with the outside world is instantaneous and automatic. It happens with the touch of thought."

– Deepak Chopra

Remember when you were a child and you would try walking on the edge of a curb without falling? Or on a high-beam or tight rope in gym class? It took balance, focus and all of your concentration, right? As the years go on, many people lose their balance, both physically and figuratively. Why does that happen?

Meet Julia. Julia is a successful businesswoman. A single mom with two teenage kids, Julia still makes time to exercise regularly and has a fairly active social life – all while spending time with her wonderful family. On the downside, Julia has been experiencing financial difficulties because she has overextended her credit and feels lonely without a romantic partner in her life. She wishes she could have better control over the things that make her unhappy, but somehow while she tries, she never achieves what she hopes for.

Although on the surface Julia's life looks pretty balanced, she lacks equilibrium. When she feels frustrated, she lays awake at night thinking about her financial difficulties. When she feels lonely, she goes shopping for a little retail therapy, which only compounds her financial distress. She's trapped herself in a vicious cycle of unhappiness and frustration.

Anne's story is only slightly different. Anne is a stay-at-home mom with three young children and a supportive, loving husband. Anne doesn't exercise much, if at all, and is overweight. As a result, Anne feels unattractive and undesirable, which contributes to a lack of intimacy in her marriage. While she has dreams of taking dance lessons and yoga classes, she feels too embarrassed to be seen in such places, due to her size. In fact, just the thought of it makes her reach out for some comfort which, surprise, she can only find in food. Do either of these scenarios sound familiar to you? Although many of us are aware of the negative behaviors in life, we're not always able to identify why we act so negatively, or more importantly, how to remedy the situation.

Remember we talked about continuing to drive when our warning light is on and how damaging and potentially dangerous that can be? Think about a car with a flat tire. If we're driving around with a flat, we won't get very far and we'll thud along the road causing even more damage to the car. Living our lives with any one area that is out of balance, will cause us to thud around and will eventually damage other areas of our life. In order to change that tire, we need to know that it's flat in the first place, we need to know how to fix it and we need to avoid whatever bump or spike in the road made it flat to begin with.

The first step in bringing balance to our lives is to bring awareness to the areas that have been neglected. Are we lacking love, self-confidence, financial freedom, peace of mind, boundaries? What areas of our lives are not quite the way we would like them to be?

Once we become aware of the areas that are lacking, we can then accept those deficiencies without judgment. It serves no purpose to blame or criticize ourselves or others for the state of our lives. By accepting and loving ourselves in spite of the negative choices we've made in the past, we are now in a position to make better choices that will direct us towards a better life. Face it, embrace it and then shift it.

In Julia's case, with the direction of a life coach, she became aware that her loneliness provoked her poor spending habits since shopping filled a void and gave her comfort. Julia learned that she needed to change her destructive habits by replacing them with more positive behaviors that would give her an opportunity to find the loving relationship she desired. Engaging in activities where she could meet new people (e.g., dance lessons, golf lessons, etc.). This step would be a good start, she discovered.

In Anne's case, she also hired a life coach and became aware of what triggered her need for comfort food. She started her customized Creating Wellness™ program and established a convenient menu plan and exercise routine that would work for her at home, while she took care of her children.

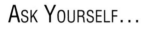

ASK YOURSELF...

- What areas of my life are off balance? Health, wellness, finances, spirituality, leisure, relationships, home, boundaries?

- What is the real cause of my imbalances?

- What am I hiding from?

- What don't I want to face?

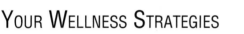

YOUR WELLNESS STRATEGIES

- Make a list of two or three areas of your life where you would like to make changes.

- Create a vision board that reflects the areas of your life, on which you want to work.

Example: I want to lose 15 pounds in the next 90 days. To do this, I will...

- Walk for 30-minutes, four times each week

- Meet with a Wellness Coach

- Follow a menu plan each day

- Exercise consistently using fun and empowering videos

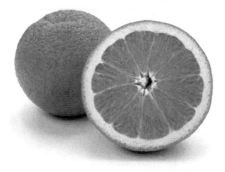

Chapter 32: Water And Your Body

– Dr. Nathalie

"Water is the only drink for a wise man."
– Walden Thoreau

I never fully realized the impact of the different sources of our drinking water and their effect on our health and well-being until I started doing research for my book. It was a serious eye opener for me and led me to make changes in my own life. Hopefully, the information you acquire from this chapter will make as big a difference in your life as it did in mine. There is a great deal of controversy surrounding the safety of tap water and the safety of bottled water. I have gathered useful facts and outlined the pros and cons on the different types of water available to us. This will help you make your own decision on the type of water you want to drink and the impact you want to make on your internal and external environment.

The role of water is nothing less than miraculous. It affects us on a number of levels and can literally make the difference between life and death.

Water's Role

- Supplies body's tissues with oxygen and nutrients
- Flushes toxins from the body
- Is essential for circulation
- Regulates the body's cooling system
- Protects cells from diseases and viruses

- Acts as a lubricant around joints
- Maintains proper muscle tone
- Improves skin tone, texture and resilience
- Is a natural diuretic
- Acts as a natural appetite suppressant
- Helps metabolize stored fat
- Is necessary for proper digestion and nutrient absorption
- Helps prevent premature aging

At birth, our bodies are made up of approximately 90 percent water, which decreases to 75 percent by the age of three. Then, as we grow older, water levels can dip to as low as 65 percent, even though our bodies are healthiest when they are well-hydrated. For most adults, the body is composed of about 70 percent water, which is recycled approximately every 15 days. Notice that it's not 70 percent coffee, tea, pop or juice! I don't know how many times I get this answer from my patients when I ask about their daily water intake: "I drink a lot of water – I have at least five coffees per day – that's water, right?" Wrong! Caffeinated beverages are actually diuretics and will dehydrate your body. Therefore, they actually increase your need to consume even more water. As for juices, you must be careful and take into consideration the sugar content and the added water needed *from* your body to dilute it during digestion. When you consume water with added flavors and ingredients, your body must work overtime to first process those substances before using the water to replenish your cells. Also be aware of the "flavored" waters with artificial sweeteners; these chemical sweeteners have been shown to be toxic and detrimental to our health.

The point is, nothing can replace our bodies' need for water and despite our bodies' water requirements, it has been estimated that 75 percent of North Americans are chronically dehydrated and fail to drink the recommended amount of at least eight cups of water (250 ml X 8) a day. In fact, studies show that the majority of people only drink about two-thirds of what they need to replace their fluid loss. Keep in mind that if you drink only when your mouth is dry and you feel thirsty, you've already put your body through dehydration.

Results of Slight Dehydration
- Premature aging
- Dry skin

- Sunken eyes
- Slowed urine production
- Kidney problems
- Dizziness
- Migraines
- Fatigue
- Indigestion/heartburn
- High blood pressure
- High cholesterol
- Arthritis
- Lupus
- Joint and back pain
- Osteoporosis
- Muscle/nerve pain
- Muscle cramping
- Excess body weight
- Diabetes
- Cancer
- Asthma
- Allergies

Keep in mind that you can lose up to 2,500 ml of water every day through urine, intestinal waste, lungs and skin. If you add other dehydrating factors such as a hot climate, exercise and dehydrating/sugary foods and beverages, your need for water increases dramatically.

Apart from water, oxygen is the only other constant bodily requirement: without it we would be dead within minutes. Without water, we could survive only a few days.

If you're not one who likes to guzzle lots of water, keep in mind that fruits and vegetables are very good sources of water. Cantaloupe and melons contain more than 90 percent, as do leafy vegetables such as lettuce. Kiwis are another great source of water and they also contain essential electrolytes such as potassium and magnesium. Be proactive in giving your body the water it needs and it will reward you in countless ways!

To find out your hydration requirement, follow one of the two methods below:

Method #1

Since the National Research Council recommends fluid intake of 1 ml/kcal per day...

- A woman on a 2,200 kcal diet would need about 2,200 ml/day; (approximately nine cups/day)

- A man on a 2,900 kcal diet would need about 2,900 ml/day. (approximately 12 cups/day)

Method #2

Another way to measure how much water you need on a daily basis is to divide your weight in pounds by two. That's how many fluid ounces you need – there are eight fluid ounces in one cup (250 ml). Add one extra cup for each hour of strenuous activity you do.

E.g. 128 lbs ÷ 2 = 64 oz (8 cups)

Water Sources

There are three main sources of water: municipally treated, well-water and bottled water.

Municipally Treated Water

- A liter of tap water in Canada costs taxpayers less than one-tenth of a cent, according to Toronto's municipal government;

- Tap water is chlorinated and sometimes fluoridated – both toxic chemicals;

- Tap water can be acidic. When consuming acidic water, our body fluids become more acidic, potentially increasing the risks of disease;

- Tap water varies depending on where you get it. For example, in some industrialized cities, municipal drinking water can have traces of lead, arsenic, asbestos, benzene, mercury, nitrites, radium, nitrites, sulfate, PCBs; radon coli form bacteria, and over 70 other contaminants. Chlorine is added to this water to kill bacteria but the dead bacteria and the chlorine still remain in the water. Chlorine has been linked to cancer, heart disease and stroke. Some people say they can also taste the chlorine in tap water due to its very distinct taste and smell;

- Fluoride is also a substance sometimes added to water in some municipalities. This is a controversial subject, since fluoride is thought to be a carcinogen (cancer-causing) and can leach the calcium from our bones;

- There are concerns that agricultural runoff adds pesticides and fertilizers to the water system;

- There are concerns of pharmaceutical (particularly estrogen) and personal care products passing through our water system;

- Tap water is stored in reservoirs and passes through piping to get to your sink. Ask yourself if you're comfortable knowing that every time you reach for your tap?

For more information on your local drinking water; go online and enter your city's name in your search engine. All cities have water quality information listed on their websites.

Well-water and Bottle

- Unmonitored system;
- Can become contaminated overnight.

The safety of well-water is entirely the responsibility of the well's owner. Given that there is no monitoring system, the safety of the water can be questionable. While well-water is supposed to be tested every six months, this water can become hazardous in just hours. If your well-water has a strange smell or taste, or if your family is developing unexplained illnesses, test your water immediately. Most cities provide free testing for privately owned wells.

Bottled Water – spring, mineral, tap or distilled water:

- Expensive – up to 3,000 percent markup;
- Creates a landfill problem – according to Canadian MacLean's magazine, May 2007, an estimated 88 percent of bottles are not recycled;
- May still contain bacteria;

- Plastic leaches toxic chemicals into the water;
- 40 percent of bottled water sold in North America is municipal filtered and treated tap water – bringing the concerns of tap water into play;
- Bottled water tends to be more acidic – disease/cancer thrive in acidic environments;
- Bottled water tends to be more deprived of natural minerals.

More and more evidence shows adverse health effects associated with the use of bottled water. A major concern is significant leaching of the toxic chemicals antimony and bisphenol-A (BPA) from certain plastic bottles. There is also a concern that washing plastic water bottles and re-using them increases the chemical leaching process. BPA may be capable of altering the normal function of genes and has also been shown to mimic the hormone estrogen and can disrupt reproductive functions. While the precise adverse health effects associated with the leaching of chemicals are uncertain at this time, it is recommended that you do not refill a plastic water bottle (single use). Also, be aware that while most beverage companies issue a two-year expiry date for unopened water bottles, it is recommended that you keep them for no more than six months.

The disagreement between the plastic industry and independent researchers relates to the fact that the plastic industry is saying that the amount of leaching is not at a dangerous level for our health. Industry studies show no harmful effects, while independently-funded research, contradicts these studies. Who to believe? Why take the chance? Why not try to minimize the risk?

Plastic Codes – What Do They Mean?

What is plastic? It's a moldable material made from petroleum. Each plastic item, including water bottles, is marked with an identification number that identifies that a particular type of plastic was used. The code is typically found on the bottom of a container and is often displayed inside a three-arrow symbol: like this <<< 3 >>>. While the codes help identify different plastics for recycling, there is still some controversy over whether they provide guidance on the safety of the plastic product being authorized for use.

Here are the categories of plastic and helpful guidelines:

Safest Plastics

- **#2 High Density Polyethylene** (HDP) – found in milk/detergent bottles, freezer bags...

- **#4 Low Density Polyethylene** (LDPE) – found in sandwich bags, bread bags...

- **#5 Polypropylene** (PP) – found in medicine bottles, cereal liners...

Questionable or Harmful Plastics

- **#1 Polyethylene Terephthalate** (PET or PETE) - found to leach antimony and BPA. Found in single use water bottles, pop, juices bottles...

- **#3 Polyvinyl Chloride** (PVC) - found to leach di-2-ethylhexyl phthalate (DEHP) and bisphenol-A (BPA), both endocrine and hormone disruptors. Found in shower curtains, meat wrap...

- **#6 Polystyrene** (PS) – may leach styrene, a possible endocrine disruptor and human carcinogen, into water and food. Found in take-out containers, foam packaging...

- **#7 PC/PLA : Polycarbonate** - this plastic is made with BPA – leaching is a huge concern. Found in baby bottles, food can liners, nylon...

From a health point of view, at the time of this writing, it is recommended to drink from the safe plastics (#2, #4 and #5), or from glass or high quality stainless steel with a metal cap. If you choose to go with aluminum, ensure that it has an inner lining.

Environmental Concerns

For years, Canadian David Suzuki and other environmentalists have spoken against the environmental evils of bottled water – the pollution generated and the energy expended in their production and the shipping is even more tragic. Despite being recyclable, plastic bottles rarely get recycled. According to a 2002 MacLean's report, Canadians alone send 65,000 tons of plastic beverage containers, many of them water bottles, to landfills or incineration establishments every year. Since plastic breaks down at a very slow rate, these plastic bottles will remain in landfills for hundreds of years to come.

Just the processing of plastics can cause serious pollution, affecting both the environment and our health. The production of one kilogram of PET plastic, which is often used for water bottles, requires 17.5 kilograms of water – which is significantly more than what those bottles themselves will contain! There is also concern related to the petroleum waste from the manufacturing of plastics.

In addition to wasting water to create water, add to that the fact that a quarter of the 89 billion liters of bottled water produced worldwide every year are consumed outside their country of production origin. That means we should also be concerned about the carbon dioxide emissions caused by transporting the bottled water since this contributes to the global problem of climate change. We keep talking about reducing our carbon footprint!

Okay, so you're probably now wondering how you're going to get your daily water requirement. Keep reading!

Bottled Water vs. Tap Water

Is one better than the other? The bottled water industry claims that bottled water is better for you than tap water, although governmental agencies such as Health Canada claim there is no evidence to support that theory.

Tap water is regulated by the Environmental Protection Agency (EPA) for hazardous chemicals, pesticides and bacteria, and is tested almost daily. Bottled water is also monitored, but under the Food and Drug Act (FDA), and while most manufacturers adhere to some EPA standards, the FDA does not mandate its testing.

For example, Toronto's tap water must meet standards for 160 contaminants, while bottled water only has standards for less than a half-dozen. And while the City of Toronto performs over 650 bacterial tests every month on its water, the extent of tests performed on bottled water is neither known nor regulated. City tap water must be filtered and disinfected. In contrast, the regulations are not as stringent for filtration or disinfection of bottled water.

Alas, the health values of all three types of water sources – tap, well and bottled – are questionable, so where should you get your water? I recommend finding a source you can *control yourself;* your own home filtration system. Filtering out the contaminants with a quality home water filtration system at the point of source, just prior to consumption, is the *best way* to be certain that you are consuming healthy water!

Water Filtration

Water treatment devices are anything but simple: carbon filters, mechanical filters, distillation units, reverse osmosis units, water softeners, iron filters and neutralizers. There are multiple treatment systems available on the market but there are three common ways to filter water – distillation, reverse osmosis and common filtration devices. It is worth the time to do your own research on filtration methods. Based on my readings, there is a great deal of information and opinions on the matter.

Distillation

Process: Distillation units boil water to create steam which is then condensed, leaving contaminants behind.

- Reduces chlorine, heavy metals, viruses and bacteria;
- Removes minerals such as nitrate, sodium, sulphate and many organic chemicals;
- Contaminants such as chloroform, a known carcinogen, will remain in the end product;
- Heating chamber must be cleaned regularly;
- Is time-consuming;
- Noisy;
- Water is depleted of minerals and long-term consumption may lead to the leaching of minerals from your body;
- Creates acidic water.

Reverse Osmosis

Process: Contaminants are removed by forcing water through a semi-permeable membrane to filter out contaminants.

- Variety of materials for membrane will impact effectiveness on different chemicals;

- Wasteful – takes at least four gallons of unprocessed water to produce one drinkable gallon of water;

- Expensive;

- Slow process;

- Water is depleted of essential minerals;

- Creates acidic water.

Activated Carbon Filters

Process: water flows through a carbon filter as contaminants are "attracted" to the positively charged and highly absorbent carbon particles.

- Activated carbon filters reduce general taste and odor problems; as well as chlorine residue;

- Activated carbon filters do not remove nitrate, bacteria or metals;

- The design of the filters greatly influences individual efficiency;

- They filter a high percentage of contaminants;

- Need to be replaced regularly;

- Cost-efficient;

- Water may be depleted of essential minerals;

- Water may be on the more acidic side due to the depleted minerals.

One sure way to take the guesswork out of a filtration device is to check if it's certified by the National Sanitation Foundation International (NSF). Certification by the NSF signifies that the manufacturer's performance claims have been validated and that the materials used in the construction of the device are safe and up to standards.

Do your due diligence when choosing a water system. Having a home filtration system gives you control over what you are drinking and is a step towards decreasing your plastic use. I recommend, for the reasons previously discussed, a high quality activated carbon filter. Portable water bottles with integrated filters are also now available. Do your research on the efficiency of the filter and remember to use a safe plastic or a high quality stainless steel bottle. These bottles are great when you don't have access to your home filtering system and are on the go. You can refill with tap water and the filter does the job!

PiMag Water – What Is It?

PiMag water was first identified in Japan over 30 years ago in a remote area surrounded by hills containing magnetite and calcium. Water was flowing over silicates, which is the material that forms natural crystals.

The Japanese discovered that the water from this stream had an amazing effect on the surrounding plants. They named it 'Pi water,' or, 'Water of life.' Then they set out to duplicate these natural conditions to spread the health benefits of their discovery.

Infusing minute amounts of ferric ions into water creates Pi water. This water also has antioxidant capabilities to help with reducing free radicals, which have a destructive effect on our bodies and cause us to age prematurely. Since Pi water also has an alkaline pH, it passes through the body's tissues more efficiently, thereby hydrating us more effectively.

The PiMag advanced filtration technologies includes several filtration stages. Adapted filtration technology reduces contaminants without adding chlorine or other chemicals to the water. Ceramics and sea coral are added to reproduce the minerals present where the Pi water was identified. Magnetic technology completes the process to reduce mineral build up and helps condition the water. I personally enjoy the PiMag Water Filtration System. For more information, you can visit www.nikken.com.

PiMag water technologies:

- Removes heavy metals and organic matter like chlorine (99.8 percent);
- Breaks down large molecules making water "wetter" – meaning it is better absorbed by the body;
- Returns essential minerals and nutrients into the water;
- Creates alkaline water, which is more in harmony with our bodies' natural fluids;
- Improves taste and odor;
- Is cost-effective.

ASK YOURSELF...

- How many glasses of water or how many liters of water do I drink every day? Is it enough?

- Where does my water come from?

- Do I know what's in my water?

- How many plastic water bottles do I use per week?

- Am I drinking from the "safe" plastic?

- Do I truly recycle every plastic water bottle I use? How about when I'm at the gym, on the bicycle path....?

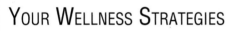

YOUR WELLNESS STRATEGIES

- Measure your daily water requirements with one of the methods mentioned in this chapter.

- List one action that you can take today to drink more water (i.e. put a glass of water on your desk to remind you to drink).

- Calculate the cost of all the bottles of water you drink in one week and then figure out how much it costs per year (x 52 weeks) and compare to the cost of a good filter and consider your carbon footprint.

- Invest in a filtration device at home and even for the office.

- Use glass, high quality stainless steel or "the safe" plastic bottles to carry your own freshly filtered water "on the go".

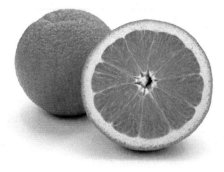

Chapter 33: Boundaries – Stop! You Are In My Space

– Andrée

"The best boundaries are loving ones."
– Dr. Henry Cloud and Dr. John Townsend

Boundaries are like fences we put up to keep others from encroaching on our space. That may sound like a selfish, uninviting thing to do, but if you think about it, it makes sense. If we didn't have boundaries, we'd let our kids steal, donate to every telemarketer who called the house or, maybe and worst of all, allow people to walk all over us. So, check in with yourself for a moment; do you ever feel taken advantage of? Do you ever feel like people don't respect you or your time or perhaps you feel people don't understand your needs? If any of these sound familiar, read on… perhaps you need to look at where you have or have not set healthy boundaries.

Simply put, boundaries signify what you decide to allow or not to allow in your life. A boundary is like an invisible line in the sand that says, "You can't cross this. It's my turf". Unfortunately, it's often easier said than done.

Many people are so programmed to accept negative, demanding behaviors from others. They are so programmed to cater to what those people want, they fail to see the freedom, empowerment and strength that can come with setting limits or boundaries. Why is that? Are they afraid of rejection, confrontation, abandonment and/or guilt? It could be all those things and more.

Here is an example of consuming guilt. John was a good son, father and husband but sometimes he got so frustrated and resentful that he felt like he could scream. When he got really frustrated, he would lose his temper with his kids and wife. When John started to meet with a life coach he complained that he had no time for himself, no life of his own and no balance in his life. He felt alone and lost. He wanted time to read a book or take a music class or just go out with the guys. All of this he thought was impossible. John had been available for his family for as long as he could remember. He never asked for time for himself, never complained to his family, but inside he was screaming to get out of his life. Because he never voiced his wants or his needs, no one around him knew what he was feeling. John had never set boundaries with anyone around him so his family took for granted that he was there to meet all their needs.

You see, we really do teach others how to treat us. From the time we're old enough to say "yes" to other people's requests, we start teaching people what we will and will not do for them.

By always complying with everyone else's wants and needs, and never making time to attend to our own, we teach others that we don't mind putting ourselves on the back burner – and that isn't healthy. The people pushing us to do this aren't necessarily selfish or inconsiderate; they simply do it because we've given them permission to by not setting boundaries. And then we begin to feel resentful, victimized and abused. It's up to you, and only you, to turn that around and set boundaries that will give us back our lives, rather than simply help others live theirs.

Time is another thing many people give away carelessly. How many times have you said, "I don't have time to exercise," "There's no time to relax," or "I have no time to read a book"? Take a magnifying glass to those statements and really explore the hours you truly have in a day and how many of them are given away to other people? Now we recognize that some days will be just like that, with work, family, friends and community responsibilities pulling you in every direction. Going to bed exhausted every night feeling resentful, is certainly not a good way to rest your body or your mind and live a healthy life. Ask yourself, is that really how you want to feel? Is this the life you really want? Think where all of this unbalanced giving leaves you and your dreams. Giving to those you love is a beautiful thing – but how can you do it for the right reasons and in the right amounts?

Remember, denying our own needs for an extended period of time will affect our well-being and that of those around us. If we're not taking time to regenerate and re-energize, eventually our mental and physical health take the hit. It might start with increased feelings of frustration, resentment and anger. It will eventually lead to stress that will break down our body and spirit.

Here are three quick steps to start you on the path of setting some solid boundaries – and not just lines in the sand that can be washed away at the first request of a friend or loved one:

- Recognize where and when you feel like you're giving away too much of your time and energy. Are you giving all your time to your family, your friends or your boss?

- Ask yourself what changes you could make to take control of your life. For example, could you talk to those around you about what your needs are?

- Start by saying "no" on occasion. Is there someone in your life who is taking too much of your time or making unreasonable requests of you? If so, be true to yourself; learn to say "no". Even if you only start with a few occasions.

It's important that you learn to say no, to set solid boundaries in your relationships, to honor your own feelings, to be at peace with your decisions and to dump guilt so that you can live life to its fullest. Look for approval only from within yourself.

ASK YOURSELF...

- What is it costing me to not have solid boundaries?

- How is my well-being affected by not having boundaries?

- What areas of my life could have better boundaries?

- What would be the reaction of friends and loved ones to my establishing boundaries?

- Do I really believe their feelings for me, or opinions of me, would negatively change?

YOUR WELLNESS STRATEGIES

- Pick one area of your life where you would like to set better boundaries – in a relationship with your partner/kids/friends/parents.

- Set one boundary this week in one area of your life. Say no to someone – someone who repeatedly takes for granted that you can run errands for them when they are perfectly capable of doing so themselves.

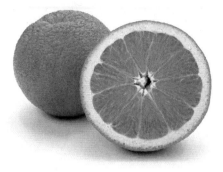

Chapter 34: Cosmetics – Painting A Different Picture

– Dr. Nathalie

"There is no cosmetic for beauty like happiness."
– Countess of Blessington

"The term 'cosmetic' means: (1) articles intended to be rubbed, poured, sprinkled, or sprayed on, introduced into, or otherwise applied to the human body or any part thereof for cleansing, beautifying, promoting attractiveness, or altering the appearance, and (2) articles intended for use as a component of any such articles; except that such term shall not include soap."
– Federal Food, Drug & Cosmetic Act (U.S.), Sec. 201 (i)

Did you know that the number one role of your skin is to act as a barrier? Even so, everything we put on our skin is absorbed and goes into our bloodstream. As a result, we shouldn't put anything on our skin that we wouldn't eat!

According to research, the average person absorbs about five pounds of cosmetic chemicals every year, and nine out of 10 women use makeup past its best-before date, thereby increasing the risk of irritation or contamination.

Take note of how many personal products and cosmetics you use every day. Here is a "typical" daily routine for most females. The alarm goes off in the morning, you jump in the shower, use shampoo, conditioner, body soap… then you get out of the shower and perhaps put on body and face cream, then comes the foundation, bronzer, eye shadow, eyeliner, mascara, lipstick routine, followed by deodorant and maybe some perfume. Throughout the day, you may re-apply some makeup, moisturize your hands, etc. Before you go to bed, you use at least one product to remove your makeup and re-moisturize. Fourteen products – see my point!?

The chemicals in your cosmetics can seep into your blood stream in a variety of ways. Take note that powders are absorbed the least, while those that are oil-based or designed to moisturize will be absorbed more. Eye makeup most certainly affects the health of the eyes – a very sensitive mucous membrane. Lipstick is often ingested. And hairspray and perfumes can irritate your lungs when inhaled.

Unfortunately, cosmetics in the U.S. and Canada are not currently regulated by an overseeing body. The cosmetics industry is, in fact, a self-regulated one, which means your safety isn't going to be a priority – sales are. It's estimated that there are about 10,500 chemicals used in cosmetics and only 11 percent of those have been tested for safety. In addition, any chemical compound created before 1970 is grandfathered and never needs to be tested for safety – it's assumed that time has been a good enough test. While some chemicals have been lightly tested and deemed to be 'Substances Generally Recognized as Safe (GRAS)'; even those chemicals haven't been studied adequately, and their long-term effects haven't been determined, nor what kind of consequences they could have when mixed with other synthetic products.

Cosmetics Hazards

There are some chemicals in cosmetics that you need to stay very clear of. These are known to be hazardous to human health. The Environmental Working Group, a non-profit organization, has created a cosmetic safety database that will help you find out safety rating of makeup, visit www. cosmeticsdatabase.com. Products are ranked from one (low hazard) to 10 (high hazard) and the site will tell you whether a product has been linked to cancer, causes allergies, is hazardous to your organs, could affect an unborn baby and more.

If you haven't found a certain product on the cosmetics database and the ingredients aren't included on your product's label, try looking up the ingredients online or even call the cosmetics company to find out. You need to know what your body is absorbing. Campaigns by organizations like the

Environmental Working Group are pushing for changes in the legislation of cosmetics to help protect you better.

The following is a list of chemicals used in cosmetics to avoid or really strive to limit:

- Lead – lipstick can contain lead, which is a neurotoxin and can cause health problems including learning, language and behavior problems;

- Aluminum – in eye shadows; has been linked to Alzheimer's disease;

- Parabens – commonly found in shampoos and deodorants to extend their shelf life. Parabens are stored in your body fat and can mimic the hormone estrogen. Parabens have also been linked to breast cancer;

- Phthalates – found in lotions and fragrances, these chemicals can be harmful to your liver, kidneys and even harm a developing fetus;

- Sodium Lauryl Sulfate (SLS) – used in skin/hair products and products that foam, this chemical is actually a harsh skin irritant that is potentially carcinogenic;

- Coal Tar – used to color products, this chemical has been linked to cancer;

- Talc – in powders, this has been shown to cause cancer in animals;

- Propylene Glycol – this is found in thousands of cosmetic products to help moisturize. It is also an ingredient used in antifreeze and brake fluid…no surprise that it may cause liver abnormalities and kidney damage;

- Polyethylene Glycol – this is used in cleansers to dissolve oil and grease. It has also been shown to be carcinogenic;

- Mineral Oil/Paraffin/Petrolatum – these are by-products of petroleum, the same stuff you put in your car. These ingredients sit on your skin and block pores by forming an oil film, creating a build-up of toxins, which may aggravate acne and promote premature aging;

- Fragrance – when you see this word on a label it can indicate the presence of up to 4,000 separate ingredients. It can also be carcinogenic and toxic.

"Natural", "Organic" or "Mineral"

Beware of cosmetic products claiming to be 'Natural', 'Organic' or 'Mineral'. They still need scrutiny. Since the terms 'organic' and 'natural' aren't regulated, it's hard to tell whether cosmetics making such claims are going to be any better for you. Look, when possible, for the certified organic logo and/or eco-certification. True natural makeup will use base products such as jojoba oil and candelilla wax instead of the petrochemicals such as mineral oil (a gasoline by-product). Mineral oil is not recommended because it will clog pores and leave an oily residue on your skin. It is also absorbed very rapidly and goes into your blood stream.

Mineral-based makeup (not to be confused with mineral oil), is gaining popularity. Minerals in cosmetics are not a new thing, they are already in most of the cosmetics you own – minerals and tons of other added chemicals. What's new, however, is that the demand for purely mineral cosmetics is growing. This kind of makeup is free of chemicals, preservatives and dyes. Since they are more granular powders, mineral-based cosmetics are minimally absorbed by the body. Dermatologists and health care practitioners also like them because they don't cause many allergic reactions; they're highly recommended to those who suffer from acne, dermatitis and other skin diseases.

Mineral makeup typically includes inorganic dyes and minerals such as mica, titanium dioxide, and iron oxide. Here's a breakdown of what those minerals are used in and where they come from:

- Titanium Dioxide – comes from the Earth's surface. Is used in foundations and is a great natural protector against UVA and UVB rays;

- Mica – comes from the Earth's surface and is used to give cosmetics sparkle and shine;

- Iron Oxide – natural salts used to add color to makeup;

- Zinc Oxide – occurs in nature as the mineral zincite. Used in creams and lotions and has broad spectrum UVA and UVB protection. Gives mineral makeup a large array of colors.

The price of mineral cosmetics isn't even that much higher than conventional ones. If you traditionally buy high-end cosmetics, you'll notice that the price is about the same or even less. Knowing, however, that you're putting something on your body that isn't hazardous to your health is priceless.

Useful Information and Links:

- Environmental Working Group www.ewg.org

- Skin Deep: Cosmetic Safety database www.cosmeticsdatabase.com

- Cosmetic Ingredients Review panel www.cir-safety.org

- www.safecosmetics.org – you can download a 'healthy cosmetics party kit' where you will find tons of useful information, resources for campaigns, contacts and even homemade recipes for face scrubs, masks etc…

ASK YOURSELF…

- What ingredients are in the cosmetics I use regularly?

- Am I influenced by the fashion industry/media into buying unhealthy cosmetics?

- How can I teach my daughters, sisters and friends to ignore the pressure tactics of the beauty industry and start to pay attention to the dangers of these ingredients?

YOUR WELLNESS STRATEGIES

- Make a list of the beauty products you use daily.

- As you do with food, read the labels on all your beauty products and cosmetics.

- Replace your regular cosmetics with safer alternatives. You can find them at your local health food store or online.

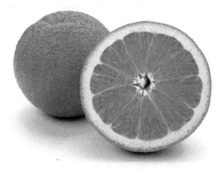

Chapter 35: Love And Intimacy

– Andrée

"Do all things with love."

– Og Mandino

If you think this is a chapter about romance and sex, think again. The kind of love you're going to read about here is the unconditional kind, an intimate connection with yourself.

Everyone has been in love – that mad, passionate love that makes you forget who you are and what your needs and wants are, because you're so focused on the feelings of euphoria that come with being in the early stages of romance, where everything is shiny and new and full of possibilities. With this kind of love, there is no logic; your heart is engaged, your brain is on hold, your emotions are jumbled and you're humming on a different frequency.

Being infatuated is wonderful for a while, however, at some point, life has to return to normal. We simply cannot sustain the kind of "suspended animation" that the falling in love state puts us in. Whether we move on to the next stage of a relationship, or we break up with the object of our affection, the falling in love stage will recede. Is this a bad thing? Absolutely not! In fact, some experts believe only then can we really begin to experience true intimacy. If you think about it, moving on to any next stage means giving up the past and moving on to the future. Everyone has been through some sort of loss in relationships...of affection, intimacy and love. You fall apart, cry, feel bad and wonder what happened. You might even lose some of your self-confidence. Why is that? It very well may be that you loved someone else more than you loved yourself and that your self-worth was tied to how the other person felt about you.

Have you ever been in love with yourself? Have you ever valued yourself as much as you value your favorite person in the world? You need to. *How much do you love yourself?* Are you number one in your life? When you love someone you take care of them. It is time to take care of you.

If you have children, you make sure they eat right, dress warmly and stay safe. You try your best to make sure they enjoy a well-balanced life that includes sports, friends, fun activities and plenty of rest. If you're in a romantic relationship, you might give up your free time to please the other, even pick up a new hobby to please him or her. You love and care therefore you give – time, energy, money and love.

How can you love yourself as much as you love others; your children, your parents, your significant other? How can you be the object of your own affection? Start by looking at areas of your life that could use a little love. Do you make well-balanced meals for your family and yet eat on the run yourself, grabbing unhealthy snacks and using the excuse that you just don't have the time? Do you forego your daily exercise routine because you're too busy at work and at home? Do you decide not to take time to meet with friends or do fun activities because your family or career demands all that you have? If any of this sounds remotely familiar, you are not putting yourself first and not loving yourself enough.

Over time, if you don't look after yourself first, you run the risk of feeling fatigued, stressed and ultimately resentful – even putting yourself at risk for serious disease. Then when illness strikes, there is nothing left for you or anybody else. To love yourself first means finding ways to take the necessary time to rest, renew and be mindful of your health and what you put into your body. In a nutshell, it means acknowledging that you are the most important person in your life. Look for ways to take time for yourself and enjoy some of that time alone.

Steps to Loving Yourself

It all starts by accepting yourself exactly the way you are. It means caring for yourself, not because you want to look good or be good for someone else but because you value yourself enough to do it for you. You won't be proud of yourself all of the time, but just think of what kinds of behaviors you accept from others and forgive because of your love for them.

The first step towards loving yourself is getting to know yourself intimately. Find out who you really are and what your needs and wants have become. It is this intimate knowledge that will build love within you. Only then, can you be true to yourself. When you get in touch with who you really are, you will also set better boundaries around you and be stronger if and when a break-up happens – because you'll still have you.

What does loving yourself have to do with your health and wellness? Well, when you love yourself, really care about yourself, you will make better choices about what you eat, the exercise you do, even the people with whom you surround yourself. When was the last time you did something really nice for yourself, truly just for you and not to please someone else? Love yourself a little more and give it a try.

Everyone needs love and affection in their lives; it's a basic human need. When this need is not met, you will constantly search for it and, perhaps, replace it with something else that only temporarily fills the void – be it food, alcohol, shopping or any number of things just to feed that need.

What is love to you? Instead of trying to find love outside of yourself, in someone or something else, start by looking within yourself. Imagine if you could give yourself the love you need, would you have more peace of mind, more satisfaction in life? You would. You will become more self-confident, less needy and much happier with life. And in response to those new positive feelings that you exude, you'll attract others with the same disposition and energy – good people who are good for you.

Love is a feeling, an emotion that scientists would say is mostly illogical. No one can debate that love is an emotion that makes you feel warm inside. Imagine feeling like that all the time. Love yourself and it will happen.

Ask Yourself...

- Do I love myself as I am?

- What can I do to love myself unconditionally, just as I am now?

- What choices can I make to assert that I do love myself?

Your Wellness Strategies

- Today, care for yourself as you would someone you love.

- Today, write yourself an appreciation note.

- This week, buy yourself a bouquet of flowers.

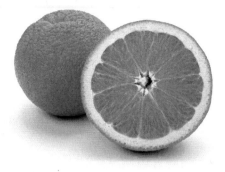

Chapter 36: It's All In The Attitude

– Andrée

"We sow our thoughts, and we reap our actions; we sow our actions, and we reap our habits; we sow our habits, and we reap our characters; we sow our characters, and we reap our destiny."

– Charles A. Hall

Your physical, emotional and mental well-being is all dependent on your attitude. Can you think of someone who went through an extremely challenging situation and unbelievable setbacks but pulled through stronger, more courageous and more successful than ever before? A person whose vision, focus and determination during the most traumatic circumstances seemed nothing less than miraculous?

Think of Oprah Winfrey, Helen Keller, Rosa Parks – they overcame huge obstacles and pushed themselves to the limit to overcome the adversity in their lives, have inspired others to do the same and have ultimately achieved tremendous success. The one attribute they had in common was their positive attitude; and that's all they needed. What they accomplished has changed the world.

Another example is Kevin Frost, a great Canadian athlete. He's won many medals worldwide in speed skating but he's no ordinary athlete. Frost is hearing-impaired and blind. He suffers from a condition called Usher's Syndrome. He lost his hearing at the age of 11 and eventually, as a young adult in his late 20s, he lost his sight.

Before losing his sight, Frost says he was a workaholic sometimes working up to 80 hours a week. He also loved refereeing hockey. His work, the refereeing, even his driver's license was taken away from him when he became blind. He could have quit life right there. But Frost, a determined father of three with the right attitude, didn't let that stop him from living. Instead, with the help of his dog Nemo who helped him adapt to his blindness, he took up speed skating, which helped release all of his pent up energy and boosted his self-confidence. Now Frost competes worldwide with able-bodied athletes. In March 2008, he competed in Germany at the World Masters Game against 280 able-bodied athletes...he ranked 18th. He also now competes with Canada's Paralympic Adaptive rowing team. What does Frost attribute his success to? Attitude! He says, "Everything happens for a reason, like it or not. But the key is to turn all negative events into positive contributions." He is certainly an inspiration.

Everyone has days when everything that can go wrong does. You wake up in a sweat because your alarm clock didn't go off, your toddler doesn't like the outfit you picked out, you spill coffee all over your favorite blouse, on your way to work there's an accident on the highway and by the time you get to work you're frazzled, your heart is racing, your breathing is shallow and now you have a headache.

Right then and there you can choose your attitude; you can choose to be miserable for the rest of the day or you can choose to let the events of your early morning go. It's a choice! You can choose how you will react to what is happening around you.

Attitude can save you. Attitude will make you laugh at yourself when you spill that coffee or provoke you to turn the radio up a little louder and sing when you're stuck in traffic. Attitude is what can prevent that headache and turn a bad day into a not so bad day. You have the choice to react to the world in a positive or a negative way. In other words, how you react to things that happen to you and around you will either make you feel good, feel confident, feel well or feel yucky. It's up to you, it's your choice – GOOD or YUCKY? What happens to you matters, but how you react to what happens, matters most.

Attitude of Gratitude

What could help you generate a positive attitude of wellness? How about being grateful for what you already have or who you are? Have you ever stopped to really reflect on all that you have and all that you are? While the positive attitude will help you see events in an optimistic light, the attitude of gratitude works concurrently to have you reflect on your life as a whole and remind you of all your past successes, all the wonderful blessings you have in your life now and how proud you ought to be of your accomplishments. So if you're feeling a little down or are having a pity party, remembering the things you are grateful for may uplift your mood. Having a positive attitude and an attitude of gratitude puts you in the best possible frame of mind and will prompt you to make the best possible choices for your life, your wellness and that of your family.

ASK YOURSELF...

- What is my attitude like now?

- How do I think a simple change in attitude could change my life?

- What am I grateful for in my life?

YOUR WELLNESS STRATEGIES

- What have you done in your life that has made you proud of yourself (e.g. graduating from university, the day your son got an award for soccer, your boss giving you recognition for a job well done)? Remind yourself of what you're grateful for every day and let yourself feel regenerated. Write it down; you will be amazed at all your accomplishments.

- Close your eyes, put your hand on your heart, and relive a moment that made you feel proud.

- Put in place an action, preferably something physical, to convert your negative thought patterns into positive ones. An example would be to put an elastic band on your wrist, and every time you have a negative thought, snap it. Your mind will respond and stop thinking like that!

"Self-pity is our worst enemy and if we yield to it, we can never do anything wise in the world."

– Helen Keller

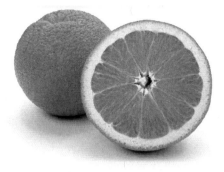

Chapter 37: Have A Ball, Really!

– Dr. Nathalie

"I have to exercise in the morning before my brain figures out what I'm doing."

– Marsha Doble

A good friend of mine who is an accomplished bodybuilder made fun of me one day at the gym for using the exercise ball to finish off my workout routine. I challenged him to give it a try! He had a quick look around to make sure nobody would see him because this was, after all, a "girly" exercise. He went flying on his first try! He couldn't even stabilize himself on the ball. It was quite funny! Now, why is it that a guy who can squat and bench press "the house" couldn't stay on that ball? It's all about the stabilizer muscles and balance.

One of the main benefits of an exercise ball – also known as a stability ball, fitness ball, Swiss ball or physio ball – is that it works multiple muscles at one time. It forces your entire body to balance itself, which engages your core muscles (abdominal, back muscles and small stabilizing muscles). For example, sitting on a bench while doing a shoulder press will work the shoulders but if you do the same exercise on a fitness ball, your core muscles are activated to keep you stabilized. Try it with pushups too – hands on the ball, even if you have to start on your knees. You will be amazed at how much more difficult simple movements can be when done on the ball.

Strengthening your core muscles will improve your overall posture and balance. Using an exercise ball as a chair at your desk is also becoming increasingly popular with office workers and students. Try using an exercise ball as a chair at work – your body will constantly be working, making small adjustments from your gluteus (buttock muscles) to your leg muscles. By doing this, you're 'actively sitting', and improving your posture with each minute instead of remaining totally sedentary. You can now find balls on wheels, which will prevent the ball from rolling all over your work area.

Our bodies are not meant to be sitting for eight to twelve hours a day, so even ergonomic desk chairs can't always promote optimal posture or prevent back slouching. Improper sitting postures can cause severe stress on the muscles, ligaments and vertebrae in your spine and consequently, on your nervous system. This can lead to headaches, migraines, neck and shoulder pain, carpal tunnel syndrome, mid and low back pain and sciatica. Integrating an exercise ball into your day or exercise routine will have a tremendous impact on your health, helping you achieve good posture, preventing back discomfort or pain and adding to your overall well-being.

An easy way to incorporate the ball into your strength training routine is to add one or two stability exercises at the end of each session. Be creative! They are not just for abdominal crunches; you can actually use them to work almost any muscle in your body. See the core strength chapter for some awesome ball exercises.

If you've never used a ball in your workout, exercise with a partner who can help you balance yourself until you get the hang of it. Or hold onto a wall or bench until you develop better balance.

What Size Ball?

The size of your ball will be determined by your height. An appropriate size ball will have you sitting with your thighs parallel to the floor, your knees at 90 degrees and your feet flat on the floor.

Height	Ball Size
Less than 5'2"	45 cm
5'2" to 5'7"	55 cm
5'8" to 6'	65 cm
6'	75 cm

Quality

The quality of the ball is also important. Ensure the material is high quality or the ball may burst, causing injury. A low quality ball will also be too soft and can't give you the support you need. This could cause you to move in a way you shouldn't or do an exercise incorrectly.

One of my patients was doing her abdominal crunches at the local gym, when the ball suddenly burst and she landed hard on her rear. Luckily, she wasn't hurt except for her pride, but she could have been badly injured. Be safe, buy quality!

ASK YOURSELF...

- How many hours a day do I spend sitting? Could I take more "active breaks" during the day?

- What is my posture like? Do I slouch? Do I feel "strong" when I'm sitting with my core muscles fully engaged?

- Could I use an exercise ball while sitting at my desk instead of a chair for a few hours per day?

YOUR WELLNESS STRATEGIES

- Purchase an exercise ball at your local fitness store. Make sure that the pump to inflate the ball is included in the kit.

- Use your exercise ball daily either sitting at your desk, watching television or to exercise.

- Be safe, start slowly by supporting yourself with a wall or another solid object. Ask the help of a personal trainer if you do not feel comfortable or safe performing ball exercises on your own.

Note: Before you attempt any exercise program, please check with your doctor.

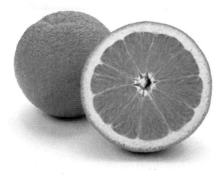

Chapter 38: Core Strength Simplified

– Dr. Nathalie

"That which we persist in doing becomes easier, not that the task itself has become easier, but that our ability to perform it has improved."
– Ralph Waldo Emerson

Stretching can be overrated! Now don't get me wrong, it is essential, but even if you are flexible enough to touch your toes, without the core strength to support your spine, you may be risking injury. My point is simply this; without core strength training, you are missing a significant component of your physical fitness.

One of my patients for example, a 45-year old man, had lower back pain for 20 years. He was fit and a runner. He had been doing stretching exercises for many years to which he was committed as part of his fitness routine. I suggested to him to suspend his stretching. He started doing core exercises as part of his fitness regimen, and when he did, his back pain went away. The stretching was harming his back because his core strength couldn't support it. Once he improved his strength, he reintroduced stretching successfully into his routine.

Core strength means keeping all those muscles required to keep your body erect, whether sitting or standing, healthy. These include the abdominal muscles, lower back muscles, hip flexors, buttock muscles, even your hamstrings and quads and also all the smaller stabilizing muscles required for good posture. Posture is the window to your spine and nervous system and is a crucial component of your well-being. Without a strong core, simple activities like reaching down to pick up a toy or bending down to unload the dryer may become problematic. A good, strong core will ultimately help you make dynamic or unilateral movements without injury.

Core Strength Exercises

The challenge with some core or abdominal exercises is that they can put a lot of stress/force on the back. There are ways, however, to achieve core and abdominal strength without harming or unnecessarily stressing your back.

Here are four core exercises you can do that will take you five minutes and will work on activating your core muscles.

1) The Front Plank
2) The Side Plank
3) The "Superperson"
4) A to Z – it's that easy!

The Front Plank

- Beginners: kneel on the floor and lean forward on your forearms keeping your spine straight. Intermediates: follow the same position but on your toes as in a push-up position. Advanced: try intermediate position while stabilizing your forearms on an exercise ball making you work harder to stay steady or you can stay on the floor and rock side to side on your forearms.

- Hold the position until you can't hold it any longer – for example when your arms or legs begin to shake. Repeat three times.

The Side Plank

- Beginners: lie down on your left side, and lift your hips and thighs off the ground by holding yourself up on your left forearm (knees are on the floor). Intermediates: take the same position but make sure you keep your knees off the floor and put your weight on your left forearm and feet. Advanced: try holding a light dumbbell and moving it around to offset the center of gravity, making you work harder.

- Hold as long as you can and repeat three times on each side. Take a 30 to 60 second break between repetitions.

The "Superperson"

- Beginners: get down on your hands and knees (like the yoga 'table position'). Lift your right arm and left leg up: hold. Make sure that your hips don't drop. Stay level from left to right with a straight back. Intermediates: use the same position on an exercise ball to increase the level of difficulty. Advanced: use the ball as intermediates, but add hand-weights and move your arm side to side while in the position to alter your center of gravity even more.

- Alternate sides and do 12 reps each side.

A to Z – It's That Easy!

- Beginners: sit on an exercise ball with your core muscles fully engaged and simply "write" the alphabet from A to Z with your hips moving back and forth and side to side. Intermediates: you can increase the challenge by holding small dumbbells in front of you while "writing" the alphabet with your hips. Advanced: as intermediates, move the dumbbells from side to side while doing your A to Z. This is also a great exercise for coordination.

ASK YOURSELF...

- Does my back hurt at the end of the day?

- Am I often sore when I bend forward or twist to perform everyday tasks?

- Do I feel I can engage my muscles when I am sitting or standing? Do I feel strong and supported when seated or saggy and awkward?

YOUR WELLNESS STRATEGIES

- Schedule two 10-15 minute sessions during your week to perform the above mentioned exercises (e.g., you could do them while watching TV).

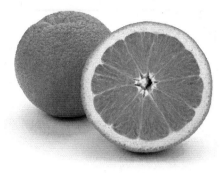

Chapter 39: Recreation Or Re-creation?

– Andrée

*"We need quiet time to examine our lives openly and honestly...
spending quiet time alone gives your mind an opportunity to renew
itself and create order."*

– Susan Taylor

Did you know that the word recreation has two very distinct meanings? The <u>Webster's Revised Unabridged Dictionary</u> defines recreation this way: refreshment of one's mind or body after work through activity that amuses or stimulates play, activity that refreshes and recreates or activity that renews your health and spirits by enjoyment and relaxation. It also defines it this way: a forming anew, a new creation or formation. Interesting!

One word, two meanings! Is it really two meanings, though? Think back to your last vacation; remember how you felt? Were you refreshed, re-energized and ready to take on the world? A break in routine, a change in daily patterns and scenery seem to give one a new outlook, a fresh start. Some of us work each year toward our vacation. We visualize where we want to go, look through brochures or websites and talk with travel agents. We plan and prepare for that all-important time when we can leave our daily routine or, for some, the daily drudgery, to enjoy our recreation time.

Now, let me bring you back to a more distant past. Remember, as a child in school, how you and all the other kids enjoyed your recreation time? The bell would ring and off you would go into the school yard with your friends to break away from the books and the lessons. After playing and chatting, most of us would go back to the classroom with a clearer head and a more focused attitude, so that we could listen to the teacher.

I remember a time, not too long ago, when 'coffee breaks' were part of the everyday office routine. We would look forward to going 'on break'. It meant breaking the pattern created by our daily work schedule; it meant chatting with friends over a coffee, building or creating relationships. Breaks were meant to re-energize and re-focus employees for the task at hand.

We all need time to re-energize and re-focus. That is why we have weekends, vacations, breaks and time-off. Much like the body needs sleep to regenerate and rebuild, the mind and spirit need a break too. Herein lies the joining of the two words; recreation and re-creation. When you are in recreation mode you have the opportunity to re-create yourself. Recreation can take many forms. Some people take a one-year sabbatical, others need only a week or two away in an exotic or foreign location and some require a 15 – 20 minute daily meditation. Whatever is needed and whatever length of time is required, the key to fully profit from recreation is to do it consciously. Recreation to re-create can simply mean resting and renewing, but it can also mean reviewing one's goals, one's career or one's purpose in life.

When was the last time you had the opportunity to re-create yourself? When was the last time you took time to look at a specific area in your life to see how you might improve it or change it? Why do we wait for a dramatic event to stop us or give us a break in order to look at our own life?

A client of mine, let's call him Peter, recently lost his job because of a merger which created re-organization in the company he worked for. For Peter, this caused incredible uncertainty and stress in his life. For the first few weeks after losing his job, Peter felt angry, confused and bitter. He went through the normal cycle of change and transition: anger, sadness and resistance.

In time, Peter came to realize that this event actually created a chance for him to explore some new and different opportunities in his career and his life. During coaching sessions, Peter expressed that he had been unhappy in his job for many years. However, with family and financial responsibilities, he felt he could not leave his job. He admitted that being pushed out of his job had given him time to reflect and review what he really wanted to do "when he grew up." While enjoying some well-deserved time off, Peter started exploring his strengths and skills, his passions and interests. Peter gained new-found self confidence that helped him see new career options ahead.

Using Recreation to Re-create Yourself!

We don't have to wait for events such as a job loss or an illness to take time and re-create ourselves. Re-creation can be a simple, daily action.

How can you better use your recreation time to re-create yourself daily? I talked in an earlier chapter about being conscious and aware in your life. That is, of course, the start of the process. Add to that a measure of playing, learning and laughing and you might just have a good recipe for re-creating yourself. Whether you want to re-create a new you, physically or psychologically, or find a new more meaningful career, using recreation to do so will generate new energy and a positive outcome.

Every day offers a new opportunity to re-create yourself. No matter where you are today, if you are unhappy or unsettled in any area of your life, you can re-create that part of your life for a whole new you.

ASK YOURSELF...

- When I take a break from my everyday life, do I take time to reflect on who I am and who I want to be?

- Do I take vacations or time off when I need it?

- What area of my life needs re-creating?

YOUR WELLNESS STRATEGIES

- Take 15 minutes in the morning to simply rest and relax. No TV, no books, just you and your thoughts. Keep your thoughts positive. If negative thoughts creep in, just notice them and then let them go, refocusing on positive thoughts. Notice how you feel afterwards.

- Use the meditation we have included in the introduction to this book or buy meditation CDs – make a decision to meditate daily. Before you meditate, ask yourself what area of your life needs a little re-creation. Simply ask the question with no expectations then start your meditation. Afterwards, take a few minutes to journal what feelings and thoughts came up for you.

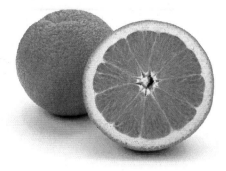

Chapter 40: Position Yourself Ergonomically

– Dr. Nathalie

"Some people like my advice so much that they frame it up on the wall instead of using it."

– Gordon R. Dickson

"My neck and shoulders are burning and my hands are getting numb at work. What is going on and what can I do?" "My back is killing me. What am I doing wrong?"

People come to my office every day with questions like these, especially if they spend their days working in front of a computer. Many of these people are suffering from what I like to call "*computeritis*" – inflammation/irritation from the computer! There is no single correct posture or arrangement of components that will fit everyone. Keep in mind that we were not designed to sit at a computer for eight to 12 hours per day. There are, however, basic design goals that everyone should consider.

In this chapter, I will provide suggestions to minimize or eliminate certain problems and allow you to create your own "custom-fit" computer workstation.

Before I can share recommendations with you, it's important to understand some basic definitions. There are two very important definitions one must understand when it comes to talking about safety and comfort in the workplace: ergonomics and repetitive strain injury (RSI). Ergonomics is the interdisciplinary study of individuals and their physical relationship with the environment in which they work. Repetitive strain injury is a general term for disorders that occur from prolonged, repetitive use of a body part which may result in pain, burning, swelling, tingling, numbness and weakness. Carpel Tunnel Syndrome is one of the most common ailments brought on by repetitive hand movements.

So who is at risk? Anyone who is performing a movement repeatedly during the day!

Improper sitting posture can create a misalignment (subluxation) in the spine causing irritation or interference with the nervous system, leading to a host of ailments, including:

- Headaches and migraines
- Neck pain
- Shoulder pain
- Carpal Tunnel Syndrome (burning in the wrists)
- Mid-back pain
- Low-back pain
- Sciatica (pain down the leg)
- Chest pain or difficulty breathing
- Digestion problems

If the ergonomics of your workstation are not designed to meet your specific body measurements or specific ergonomic needs, you *will* experience pain and that is not a healthy, positive way to spend any amount of time. Another point to keep in mind is that even if you have the Cadillac of ergonomic workstations, you're still at risk of overusing your muscles if you're there too long! So monitor the time you spend in front of the computer; get up and move on a regular basis. Try to do so every 30 minutes. If you drink a lot of water – which is a good thing for you – your body will remind you to get up!

Here are some things that you can do to personalize your computer workstation and minimize problems caused by one that is not ergonomically designed:

Set-up Your Chair

This is perhaps the most important part of designing an ergonomic workstation. The office chair should adapt to whoever uses it, not vice versa. The height, lumbar area (for lower back), armrests and depth should all be adjustable. The seat should also be firm but comfortable; the chair should have strong, sturdy wheels that allow your body to remain stable while moving around. As an option, you can always use an exercise ball as your office chair!

Guidelines:

- Modify your seat height so your feet rest flat on the floor;

- Adjust the height of your seat's backrest so the lumbar support sits in the small of your lower back;

- Ensure your shoulders are in line with your hips when sitting;

- Make sure the seat depth doesn't put pressure behind your knees when sitting against the backrest;

- Check that your armrest is adjusted so your shoulders are resting comfortably;

- Get up often!!

Adjust Your Posture

One of the easiest ways to make sure that you are sitting properly is to follow the 90-degree rule!

Guidelines:

- Your knees should be at a 90-degree angle, with thighs parallel to the floor and lower legs perpendicular;

- Your feet should rest flat on the floor and if they don't, ensure they're supported by a stable footrest;

- Your arms should be at a 90-degree angle parallel to the floor, if your armrest is too high or too low your shoulders will feel strained;

- Keep your upper arms and elbows close to your body;

- Your wrists and hands should be straight, the palm-rest should only be used between typing periods;

- Your neck should be in a neutral position or 15-degrees downward.

Adjust Your Computer Monitor

Guidelines:

- Minimize the glare on your monitor from direct light and reflections by using a screen filter;
- Leave 40 – 60 centimeters of distance between you and the monitor, about arm's reach;
- Adjust the brightness/contrast so you don't have to move to see it properly;
- Position monitor directly in front of you so you don't have to rotate your head;
- Increase font size or page view size to avoid eye strain.

Use Your Mouse and Mouse Pad Properly

- Hold mouse lightly;
- Mouse should be at the same level as the keyboard to avoid over-reaching;
- If a mouse strains your wrist too much, consider a trackball as an alternative;
- Find a mouse that is comfortable for you;
- If you're experiencing an RSI with one wrist, try changing the mouse to the other side of the keyboard;
- Try a padded mouse pad which may relieve some pressure on your wrist. Be careful that it does not press on your wrist and end up creating irritation (carpal tunnel).

Other Tips

- If you are right-handed, consider switching to a left-handed keyboard. These have the number keypad on the left side, which allows you to better center your alpha keys and bring your mouse closer to center. If left-handed, switch to right-handed keyboard;
- Don't pound on the keyboard, use a light touch when typing;

- Take breaks from typing, varying your activities as much as you can;

- If you have an RSI, try to eliminate unnecessary computer usage;

- Evaluate other activities that you do that may be contributing to your RSI;

- Always pay attention to your body's complaints – it's telling you something;

- Kids are at risk for RSIs too, so monitor their computer use. If they don't have their own computer, make sure to modify the family work station accordingly.

Exercise Tips

- Perform neck, arm and lower back stretches every hour – program your computer for reminders. Computer applications can be found online for stretching purposes;

- Incorporate ball/core exercises to improve your overall musculature and engage your stabilizing (abdominal) muscles;

- Perform aerobic exercises to help maintain a better energy level and compensate for a sedentary job;

- Perform regular strength-training exercises to ensure that your musculature is kept strong and balanced and can respond to the muscular demands of a time-lengthy position.

If, after following all the above-mentioned guidelines, you are still experiencing some discomfort or pain, I would strongly suggest talking to your employer about having an ergonomic assessment to maximize your body mechanics and prevent injury. If you are experiencing any body signals, please talk to your Wellness Chiropractor, physiotherapist or massage therapist to get a proper diagnosis of your condition and to receive proper care. Don't just ignore the symptoms or mask them! Go to the source of the problem.

Ask Yourself...

- Am I experiencing any of the body signals mentioned in this chapter? If yes, which ones?

- How ergonomic is my workstation?

- Have I had an ergonomic assessment of my workstation?

- How is my computer set up at home? Is it functional for the entire family?

- Have I consulted a Wellness Chiropractor to improve my spinal biomechanics and to ensure a fully functioning spine and nervous system?

Your Wellness Strategies

- Self-assess your workstation at work and at home to ensure that it is as ergonomic as possible, following the suggestions in this chapter.

- Commit to doing a core exercise suggested in this book at least every other day, join a gym, or do yoga to obtain postural muscle strength flexibility and to ensure that your core strength is supporting your spine and your overall well-being.

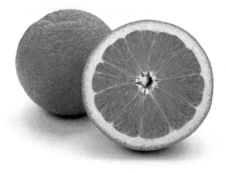

Chapter 41: Magnetism – What It Means To Us

– Dr. Nathalie

"Minds are like parachutes; they function only when they are open."
– Unknown

This chapter brings us to controversial terrain since magnetism is a topic that is often misunderstood. As a result, there are many conflicting views when it comes to the field of magnetism as it relates to health. Even for people who support the use of magnets, there are differing opinions related to design, strength and the quality of magnets, as well as the use of their poles.

In this chapter you'll learn that human beings are in fact magnetic beings and that we are surrounded by electromagnetic fields that significantly influence our health – positively and negatively.

Positive Sources of Magnetism

Magnetism is a universal force. Science has established beyond all doubt that all living cells are electromagnetic by nature, and that there are two natural sources of magnetism available to us – the Earth and our brain.

The Earth is meant to provide a steady magnetic field that our bodies can draw on to enhance molecular reactions. Scientists, however, have recorded a decline in the strength of the Earth's magnetic field over the last 165 years. Today the magnetic field of the Earth is about 0.5 Gauss, while

4,000 years ago, it's estimated that it was approximately 5.0 Gauss. This is a significant decline.

Our brain cells have the capacity to generate electricity and produce a pulsed, electro-magnetic field with efficiency. The brain and the Earth's magnetic fields work together to accomplish what is called "magnetic resonance." Magnetic resonance occurs when the brain's pulsed magnetic frequency matches the frequencies of various tissues and organs, helping to repair damaged cells, make enzymes, and enhance immunity. Since the Earth's magnetic field is depleted, our bodies are not always able to achieve the magnetic resonance necessary to restore and rejuvenate our organs and tissues. Think about it....living or working in high-rise buildings and being surrounded by concrete in big cities does affect our ability to connect with the Earth's natural magnetism. Also, the reduction in the Earth's field is the most logical explanation for the human body's positive reaction to engineered forms of beneficial magnetism – we are, often times, in a state of deficiency!

Negative Sources of Magnetism

It is quite common for people to confuse natural sources of magnetism with electromagnetic fields like power lines, cell phones, and microwaves. Electromagnetic fields (EMF) are different. EMFs have a much higher and harmful frequency, and pollute our air, water and food.

In this technological age, the negative electromagnetic frequencies our bodies are exposed to are higher and stronger than ever. The frequencies in electricity, for example, override the magnetic resonance function in your brain, impeding your organs and tissues from being repaired by beneficial magnetism and contributing to the development of chronic ailments. Even sleeping beside an electrical appliance like an alarm clock can disturb your magnetic resonance. With electromagnetic fields comes electromagnetic stress – which is just as harmful to your body as any other physical stress, even though this stress is less obvious to us. Does this sound like science fiction? Think again! Research tells us the importance of being aware of the negative impacts of electromagnetic sources.

The truth is that electromagnetism is part of our modern life and some exposure can't be avoided – no one can say they are not exposed to at least a few electromagnetic stresses throughout the day. Here are a few things you can do to decrease your exposure to negative electromagnetic fields:

- Avoid buying a house near a power site;

- Avoid unnecessary computer usage – they emit electromagnetic fields from all sides;

- Avoid carrying your cell phone or personal assistant device on your person all day;

- Use your cell phone on speakerphone when possible;

- Find a headset that offers electromagnetic radiation reduction (air tube). Do your research on this one as some technologies will emit even more radiation;

- Choose a device with the lowest SAR possible (SAR = specific absorption rate) that measures the strength of the magnetic field absorbed by the body. SAR rankings are available online;

- Avoid sleeping with an electric blanket;

- Avoid being in an environment of fluorescent light all day – incandescent light is much less harmful;

- Limit your use of a microwave oven as it may even affect the molecules of the food you eat. If you do, use safe materials like glass to microwave your food;

- Limit your TV use and avoid sleeping in front of one all night;

- Limit your use of personal appliances such as electric razors and hairdryers.

Potential Health Benefits

There is nothing new about the idea that magnets have the ability to promote healing. They've been used in this capacity for hundreds of years. Despite this, magnetic therapy is considered an alternative therapy and no medical claims can officially be made relating to its benefits. Nevertheless, there are many studies that show the positive effect of magnets on: fibromyalgia, diabetic neuropathy, cancer, multiple sclerosis, arthritis, blood circulation, general healing and post operative-recovery, and sleep.

A magnet is made up of one positive and one negative pole – North and South. Since each pole attracts molecules with an opposing charge, and since our bodies are made up of molecules that are both positively and negatively charged, it is believed that a magnet on our body can lead to improved blood flow. By improving blood flow, our cells are better able to absorb oxygen, get access to more essential nutrients, clear the body of toxic waste, and speed up the repair of damaged tissues. Besides increasing blood circulation, other theories on why magnets benefit the body include: having an effect on iron in the blood, altering the body's pH balance, improving electrical conductivity of cells, and stimulating new cell growth.

Not all magnets are created equal. Design is of utmost importance. For example, simple magnets show the flux lines (energy) around the center of the magnet, however, the surface of the top and bottom are without magnetic energy. The key is to use a design that includes the entire surface area. Some magnets on the market have a linear or circle type design. The best design allows for the number of positive and negative poles to create lines crossing the surface in order to maximize energy flow. This is called the equilateral design and means that equal-length sides and angles create a consistent magnetic field over the entire surface (Nikken® magnets are made with an equilateral design. For more information, go to www.nikken.com). Refrigerator magnets are mostly linear, and, therefore are not beneficial to the human body. These are mainly between 35 and 200 G, while magnets for the management of pain are usually between 300 and 5,000G. The equilateral design offers maximum penetration thereby providing more health benefits. Magnet quality does matter, so do your research!

Magnets can be another form of therapy that does not require drugs or surgery. Health professionals are starting to include them in their tool kits to help people in a non-invasive and non-toxic way. Athletes who require optimal performance and fast recovery from injuries can also benefit from the use of magnets.

Who should not be using magnets? Pregnant women, people who use a medical device such as a pacemaker, defibrillator, or insulin pump and even people who use a patch that delivers medication through the skin, since magnets may cause dilation of blood vessels, which could affect the delivery of the medicine. Consult your natural health care provider.

Magnetic Sleep Systems

Magnetic sleep technologies might be relatively new to the Western world but the Japanese have been sleeping on magnetic beds for years. Because the Earth's magnetic field has decreased, the idea behind a magnetic bed is to restore or recharge your body. There are several companies with a variety of magnetic products. Some are beneficial and some are not. It's important that you assess the quality of the products before you invest in it. Nikken® is one of the most popular and reputable companies that sell magnetic sleep systems designed to re-create the Earth's magnetic field. The magnets used are approximately 150 Gauss at the surface. Their magnetic field diminishes very quickly with the distance from the body so that by the time it hits your body there is only the required magnetic energy left (5 Gauss like the Earth used to be). The way I explain the concept to my patients, is that sleeping on a magnetic bed is like recharging their bodies the way they recharge their cell phone batteries every night. Be wary of magnetic beds with up to 1,200 Gauss – you do not need that much and they can do more harm than good.

Magnetic sleep systems also affect the pineal gland in your brain. The pineal gland is one of the most magnetic-sensitive glands in your body; it also produces melatonin, a hormone that helps regulate sleeping patterns. Studies have shown that when people use magnetic pads, their pineal gland is stimulated and they experience improved sleep.

ASK YOURSELF...

- How many hours per day am I exposed to electromagnetic fields?

- What can I do to decrease my daily exposure to electromagnetic fields at home or at work?

- How much time do I spend in high rise buildings away from the Earth's magnetic field?

Your Wellness Strategies

- Do an inventory of the electromagnetic fields that you're bombarded with:

  - ✓ Cell phones or personal assistant devices
  - ✓ Fluorescent lights
  - ✓ High voltage power lines
  - ✓ Microwave ovens
  - ✓ Televisions
  - ✓ Computers
  - ✓ Personal appliances

- Find a strategy which would reduce your exposure to EMFs this week (e.g. turning off the TV instead of falling asleep in front of it all night, using your speaker phone on your cell more often or acquiring a safe headset).

- Consider contacting a Natural Health Care Professional who can help you strategize about options to decrease your exposure to electromagnetic fields and "recharge" your body while you sleep.

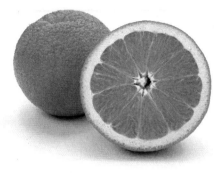

Chapter 42: Time Is On Your Side

– Andrée

"Carpe Diem! Seize the Day."

Oftentimes, people struggle with how they're going to manage their time and how they're going to fit in everything they want to do in a day. Many people feel that in their day-to-day lives they're forever running, forever catching up, and still behind in what they want to achieve. From jobs, to errands, to children, to housework – it seems to never end.

Most of us have woken up at 3:00 a.m. thinking of all the things we should have done the day before then panic about fitting it all in the next day. With this busy lifestyle, however, many people have forgotten about something absolutely crucial – themselves and what they value most.

A couple of decades ago, I worked as a training consultant for a great personal development company. I was certified to lead a workshop on value-based time management. In teaching this program, I learned as much about myself, and for myself, as did the people who attended the workshop. The philosophy behind what I was teaching was that once you identified what you value, you would use your time more productively and effectively and you would be more balanced. I loved teaching the program because I knew I was making a difference in people's lives, and, as I said earlier, it also taught me a lot about my own values and my own priorities. Let me share with you what happened.

I loved the training I was providing. I had always wanted to be a trainer. At that time in my life I was a single mom with a beautiful boy of three. I was traveling quite a bit, which, prior to being a single mom, was not an issue. Here I was raising this little kid on my own, doing work I loved, for a company whose values I shared and traveling all over the place. I was traveling to Europe, the U.S. and various parts of Canada which meant carting my little bundle of joy to various sitters while I was away. When I was traveling, I would go back to my hotel room at night and cry myself to sleep because I missed my son so much. I kid you not, it was tearing me apart. I realized I was not living my truth, not living within my own values. I was not spending my time in a way that matched my priorities.

My values had changed when my son was born. Now I was a mom and that, my friends, was my most important value. It finally occurred to me that I had to make a choice about how and where I spent my time. I had a very big decision to make, as you can well understand. So I put a plan in place, a goal of sorts, with a set time frame and eventually left my job and found a lower paying job, locally. Was it difficult? Of course! Would I do it all again? Yes! Did I have to change my lifestyle? Yes, of course. But that is what making conscious choices and real changes is all about. In the end, changing my work to fit my values, made my life so much easier and less stressful. I was able to see my baby every evening, be with him in the morning and take him to day care. I was able to sleep at night. My weekends were more relaxed because I wasn't trying to cram everything into two days before heading off once again. I was being true to myself and to my values and created a plan and daily activities to match.

So you ask, "How does that apply to me?" How can you make the most of your days, nights, weekends; your time, basically? Let's be clear here, we all have the same amount of time. I have 24 hours per day, you have 24 hours per day, so do your neighbors, your friends and so on and so on. What we choose to do with those 24 hours per day is the key. So let's leave out the seven to eight hours of sleep (and I do hope you are getting enough sleep), so that leaves you 16 hours to play with, so to speak. What you do with those hours will depend on what you value, what you think is most important to you, what your vision is and what goals you want to put in place to achieve that vision. So what is most important to you? Is it your health, your family, your friendships, your finances, your community, the environment or maybe your career?

How do you connect with what's most important? At different times in your life, different areas of your life will be more and less important, so get clear with what you value right now and prioritize your time accordingly. Look for the area in your life where you feel the most frustration or disappointment. As we saw in the chapter on awareness, being in touch with how you feel and coming face-to-face with what is not quite right is the first step to creating changes and achieving that spectacular life you are waiting to live. It's about making every day, every moment count by focusing on what is important to you.

Let's look at Pam's life for a moment: Pam, a successful bank manager, really values her health and well-being. Unfortunately, over the last couple of years she's gone through a painful divorce and has also had to care for her elderly mother. She's also raising her two teenage daughters. She could be a typical "sandwich" generation individual. Pam hasn't spent much time looking after herself; she fails to eat right or exercise because she feels she just can't spare the time, racing from one appointment to a soccer game or finishing a report for work. As a result of ignoring herself, Pam has put on weight, isn't sleeping well and has little or no energy to do any of the things she loves. Although she knows the importance of being fit and active and wants to improve that area of her life, Pam is not living according to her value of living a healthy lifestyle. Sound familiar? You are probably thinking, "Been there done that, but there is no way to change it". As difficult as it might seem, if Pam doesn't take ownership of her health and wellness, at some point, she may get ill and not be able to look after those she loves.

Pam certainly felt the tearing apart inside and just did not know how to go about making changes on her own. She felt she needed help, needed support. For Pam, hiring a life coach was the first step in making changes in her life and getting the support she needed when she felt she was about to give up on her goal. With her coach's support, Pam set out on the road to getting back into shape, back to her optimum weight and having more energy to do things she loves to do. She wants to fit into her favorite dress, something she has not been able to do for some time now. Although her final goal is set for a year from now, Pam knows that she needs to set short term goals as well as daily activities to keep her on track.

The key to reaching a goal, any goal, is to keep it foremost in your mind. How can you do that? Creating a vision board will give you the daily visual reminder of your goals. Add to that an action plan of tasks or activities in which you will engage to realize your vision. Pam's vision board included a picture of a fit and trim woman in a yoga pose, another of a group of women doing a walk for charity. Her daily action list includes activities such as walking for 20 to 30 minutes every day, preparing healthy meals ahead of time to remove the guess work of what to have for lunch. What else could she have on her list? Well, perhaps engaging her daughters in meal preparation or in helping with her elderly mom. Other actions could be:

- Research various fitness centers
- Talk to a nutritionist
- Look at meal plans
- Talk to friends about her goals

Once the action plan is set, it is time to get going! No matter how exciting your vision is, if you don't take action, nothing will happen. Pam feels good for taking the first steps towards her vision. She will notice rapidly that her self-confidence will soar because she is honoring her promise to herself.

I challenge you to start using a daily list to accomplish what you want. List up to nine things that you want to do in a day that will bring you closer to your values and your vision of a fulfilling life, whether it's changing jobs as I did, or getting fit like Pam. Whatever it is, honor yourself. At the end of each day review your list, see how many activities you have completed that are in line with your vision. Celebrate your successes, notice your setbacks without judgment, and take corrective action when you need to…without beating yourself up. The spirit with which you treat yourself as you move toward your goal will help you move forward.

Have a look at your daily activities. Are they related directly to what is most important to you? Are you putting your values first?

Ask Yourself...

- Looking at the different areas of my life, what do I value most right now – my health, career, family or friends?

- What in my life needs polishing the most?

- Do I have a one-year vision for the area of my life I want to work on the most?

Your Wellness Strategies

- Develop goals for the one area of your life you want to work on.

- List the things you need to do to meet your goals.

- Create a daily list of tasks you need to do to meet your goals.

- Create a "Purpose on the Go!" business card as a daily reminder of why you're working hard to achieve your goals.

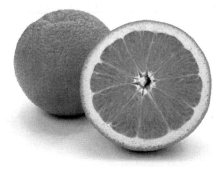

Chapter 43: Beauty Sleep

– Dr. Nathalie

"Sleep is the golden chain that ties health and our bodies together."
⌐ Thomas Dekker

Trouble sleeping? You're not alone. An estimated 3.3 million Canadians aged 15 and older, or about one in every seven, have problems getting to sleep or staying asleep – contributing to insomnia.

Part of the problem is 80 percent of North Americans say they believe it's not possible to sleep enough and be successful at their jobs. As a result, 75 percent experience daytime sleepiness and 34 percent say sleepiness interferes with their daytime activities – that's certainly no way to live.

Sleep is important for a multitude of reasons but mainly to rebuild, repair and recharge your body. When you're asleep, your immune system is most active and repairs what it needs to while your brain re-organizes your cerebral 'files'. Without sleep, you get sick in both mind and body.

Symptoms of Sleep Deficit

- Daytime fatigue
- Poor memory, mental performance
- Irritability
- Depression, apathy
- Morning headache, wake-up feeling un-refreshed

- Heart disease
- Heartburn
- Need to urinate in the middle of the night
- Loud snoring
- Diminished sex drive
- Decreased exercise tolerance
- More than five pounds of weight gain in the past year
- Need for stimulants

Why Your Body Needs Sleep

Regulates Hormones and Prevents Cancer

Lack of sleep affects hormone levels. A disrupted circadian rhythm (sleep/wake cycle) may create shifts in hormones like melatonin. Melatonin is made in the brain by converting tryptophan into serotonin and then into melatonin, which is released at night by the pineal gland in the brain to induce and maintain sleep. Melatonin is also an antioxidant that helps suppress harmful free radicals in the body and slows the production of estrogens, which may activate cancer.

A link between cancer and the disrupted circadian rhythm lies with a hormone called cortisol, which normally reaches peak levels at dawn then declines throughout the day. When you don't sleep enough, your cortisol levels don't peak as they should. Cortisol is one of many hormones that help regulate immune system activity, including natural-killer cells that help the body battle cancer.

Heart Attack and Stroke

Lack of sleep has been associated with high blood pressure and high cholesterol, both potential risk factors for heart disease and stroke. Your heart will be healthier if you get between seven and nine hours of sleep each night.

Stress

When your body is sleep-deficient, it goes into a state of stress – creating an increase in blood pressure and production of stress hormones. The stress hormones unfortunately make it even harder for you to sleep. Since reducing stress will allow your body to get a more restful sleep, learn relaxation techniques that will help counter the effects of stress.

Inflammation

When you don't get enough sleep, the level of inflammation in your body also rises. Inflammation is thought to be one of the main causes of the body's deterioration, creating more risk for heart conditions, as well as cancer and diabetes.

Energy level

A good night's sleep makes you energized and alert the next day. Being engaged and active not only feels great, it increases your chances for another good night's sleep. When you wake up feeling refreshed, and you use that energy to get out into the daylight, be active and engaged in your world, you sleep better that night.

Memory

Researchers don't fully understand why we sleep and dream but a process called 'memory consolidation' occurs while we sleep. While your body may be resting, your brain is busy processing your day and making connections between events, sensory input, feelings and memories. Getting a good night's sleep will help you remember and process things better.

Weight

Researchers have found that people who sleep less than seven hours per night are more likely to be overweight or obese. It's believed that the lack of sleep impacts the balance of hormones in the body that affect appetite. The hormones ghrelin and leptin, important for the regulation of appetite, have been found to be disrupted by lack of sleep.

Depression

Sleep impacts many of the chemicals in your body, including serotonin. People with a deficiency in serotonin are more likely to suffer from depression. You can help prevent depression by making sure you are getting the right amount of sleep.

Body Repair

Sleep is time for your body to repair damage – everything from a wound to a sunburn. Your cells produce more protein while you're sleeping and proteins are the building blocks for your cells, allowing them to repair damage.

Ways to Maximize Your Sleep

- *Listen to white noise or relaxing music*

Some people find the sound of white noise or nature sounds such as the ocean or forest to be soothing for sleep.

- *Avoid before-bed snacks*

Avoid grains and sugar. These foods will raise blood sugar and inhibit sleep. If you have to snack, choose a high-protein option, such as a whey protein shake. This will provide L-tryptophan, needed to produce serotonin and melatonin, which actually help you sleep.

- *Keep a schedule*

Go to bed and wake up at the same time every day. This will train your body to sleep on a schedule. If you can maintain this schedule for three weeks, you'll probably find yourself falling asleep faster and feeling more refreshed. To achieve this, however, you can't sleep in on weekends or stay up too late, either. Keep in mind that the natural human biorhythm is to sleep between 10 p.m. and 6 a.m.

- *Create a bedtime routine*

Create a nightly routine to tell your body that it's time to sleep. Start about 30 minutes before you lay down to help release stressful thoughts. Your routine could include meditation, deep breathing, reading or a warm bath. The key is to find something that makes you feel relaxed, then repeat it each night to help you release the day's tensions. Avoid watching TV or reading something too adventurous though, as this will stimulate your brain and likely have just the opposite effect, provoking you to stay up later.

- *Maintain a healthy weight*

Being overweight can increase the risk of sleep apnea, which will prevent a restful night's sleep. In one study, individuals who were extremely obese with a Body Mass Index (BMI) of 35 or more, had higher odds of reporting insomnia than those of normal weight, BMI of 18.5 to 24.9 (see chapter #19 – "Measure Up!").

- *Exercise daily*

Daily exercise has been shown to improve your chances of falling asleep quickly and sleeping soundly. Research shows that you get a better sleep with regular exercise. Try to exercise early in the day and avoid exercising within three hours of bedtime. Exercising too late in the day can make it difficult for you to fall asleep because it is a stimulant.

- *Make your bedroom dark*

As mentioned earlier, you need to produce the hormones serotonin and melatonin in order to sleep deeply. Since even a little bit of light will diminish their efficiency, sleep in a dark room and don't turn on the lights at any time during the night if you need to get up. Consider getting an eye mask to help you block out any light that might impede your sleep.

- *Get some sunshine*

Sunlight helps regulate your internal clock stimulating your body to produce melatonin – which normalizes your sleep cycle. You need exposure to bright light every day. Morning sunlight exposure can be especially helpful. Be sure to open the drapes every morning to let light in. Spend time outside!

- *Avoid caffeine after noon*

Some people are caffeine-sensitive and can't drink coffee, tea or any other caffeinated beverage up to six hours before bedtime. Some people just can't metabolize caffeine efficiently. If you're having trouble sleeping try to avoid all afternoon and evening caffeine.

- *Journaling*

If you often lay in bed with your mind racing, it might be helpful keep a journal and write down your thoughts before bed. This allows your mind to rest and may even help create solutions in your sleep!

- *Go to bed early*

Many of your body's systems do the majority of their recharging and recovering between 11 p.m. and 1 a.m. For example, your gallbladder dumps toxins during this time. If you're awake however, the toxins may back up into the liver, which will impact your health.

- *Avoid Alcohol*

That small glass of wine can actually make it more difficult for you to stay asleep. After an evening drink you might fall asleep just fine but you will likely wake up in the middle of the night. This effect is caused by a rebound in blood sugar and withdrawal from the alcohol after it has metabolized. Try avoiding alcohol before sleep and see if you sleep more soundly. For every drink you have, give your body at least an hour before trying to fall asleep. Keep in mind that alcohol will also keep you from falling into the deeper stages of sleep, when the body does most of its healing.

- *Be smoke-free*

The nicotine in cigarettes is a stimulant that will keep you awake – just one of the many bad things smoking does to your body. Smokers may also wake up prematurely due to nicotine withdrawal.

- *Remove the clock from view*

It will only add to your worry when you constantly watch it, so put the clock somewhere you can't stare at it all night. Also the electromagnetic frequency emitted by your alarm clock can interfere with your body's recuperating abilities as well.

- *Make preparations for the next day*

Before heading to bed, determine what you'd like to accomplish for the next day so you don't have to think about it while trying to get to sleep.

- *Invest in a magnetic sleep system*

A high quality magnetic sleep system can help your body "recharge" its own magnetic energy. The magnetism will help you get a deeper and more regenerative sleep, while helping ailments like a sore back or achy joints (see chapter #41 – "Magnetism – What It Means To Us").

- *Power naps*

If you have the opportunity, napping during the day isn't only an effective and refreshing alternative to caffeine, it also promotes wellness and makes you more productive. Studies show that people who nap several times a week have a lower risk of dying from heart disease. Napping also improves memory, cognitive function and mood.

- *See your Wellness Chiropractor*

Having an optimal spine and nervous system is very important in order to get proper sleep. Your nervous system is your body's master system and affects all your cells, tissues and organs. If you have interferences on your nervous system due to spinal misalignments caused by physical, psychological and biochemical stresses; it will have a major impact on your sleep and your body's ability to recuperate.

ASK YOURSELF...

- Am I getting enough sleep?

- Do I feel refreshed when I get up in the morning?

- Am I regularly experiencing some of the signs and symptoms of sleep deficit mentioned in this chapter?

- What behaviors or habits could I change to improve the quality of my sleep?

YOUR WELLNESS STRATEGIES

- List three behaviors that you can change this week to improve the quality of your sleep. Do this for four consecutive weeks. Experience the difference!

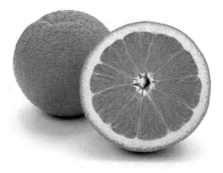

Chapter 44: Cookware Awareness

– Dr. Nathalie

"In all affairs it's a healthy thing now and then to hang a question mark on the things you have long taken for granted."

– Bertrand Russell

How safe are your cookware and cooking methods? Have you ever thought about it? Here are a few facts that you should be aware of for your safety and the safety of your family.

Pots, pans and other cookware are made from a variety of materials that can be absorbed by food when heated. Food can even react to some containers when cold. Have you ever noticed that your favorite food tastes like plastic after being stored in a plastic container? The fact is that food ions react with plastic, synthetic and even metallic ions. Temperature affects reactivity so hot food will react with a container more quickly. Refrigeration deters the uptake of metal or plastic ions.

Some foods are more reactive than others. Fat, acidic ingredients and water absorb more from containers than do proteins and carbohydrates. This explains why high quality oils, vinegar and wine are sold exclusively in non-reactive glass containers.

Questionable Choices

Non-stick Teflon

Teflon is the most popular cookware but unfortunately it contains perfluorooctanoic acid (PFOA), a synthetic chemical with major health risks linked to it. Teflon can chip off a cooking pan and get into your food.

Aluminum Cookware

Aluminum is a lightweight product that conducts heat well and is fairly inexpensive, but it's also a suspected factor in Alzheimer's disease. The World Health Organization estimates that you can consume 50 milligrams of aluminum a day without enduring harm but it's difficult (almost impossible) to measure the quantities you ingest from the products you use – and the longer food is cooked or stored in aluminum, the more it gets into your food. Green leafy vegetables and acidic foods like tomatoes will absorb the most.

Plastic Cookware

As noted previously, plastics are also a concern. The softer (more flexible) the plastic, the more apt it is to react with food and beverages. Microwaving increases the reactivity of plastics and food. And since we are often in a hurry and just want to "nuke, grab and go", we are regularly exposing ourselves to dioxins, which are carcinogens. It is best to microwave your food in glass or ceramic containers. So even if the instructions say it's safe to microwave in the plastic store-bought container, take the extra few seconds and switch to a dinner plate.

Better Choices

Stainless Steel

Stainless steel is a better cookware choice but still contains iron, nickel and chromium that can be harmful to your health. Contrary to popular belief, stainless steel may not be a completely inert metal. It's not recommended to store foods that are highly acidic in such containers. Once a stainless steel container has been scratched, even through normal scouring, the leaching of metals is higher. Look for a high quality, heavy duty stainless steel.

Silicone

Silicone is a synthetic rubber that contains bonded silicon – a natural element that is abundant in sand, rock, and oxygen. Silicone cookware is non-stick and stain-resistant, inert and safe up to 428 degrees Fahrenheit (220 Celsius). If heated above its safe range, silicon melts but does not give off toxic vapors. There are no known health hazards associated with silicone cookware at this time and it does not react with food or beverages.

Cast-iron

Cast-iron is also a good choice of cookware, because it reacts very little when heated and is less harmful to your health. One disadvantage is the weight of the cookware.

Enamel-glass and Ceramic

There's good reason why glass and ceramic beakers are used in chemistry labs – it's because they are non-reactive.

Enamel-based cookware has a fused-glass surface. With proper care, a fine enamel pot can last a lifetime, but inexpensive enamel cookware will only have a thin enamel layer. Cheap enamel cookware will chip easily and the fragments will find their way into your food.

Ceramic based cookware is non-reactive and offers the most effective heat for cooking. With ceramic cookware, the most subtle flavors emerge because there is no leaching from the container. Be aware, however, that antique ceramic may contain lead – better to buy new.

A recommended cookware product recently on the market, is the Mercola Healthy Cookware (www.mercola.com). It is not made of Teflon or other non-stick brands using perfluorooctanoic acid (PFOA) and is made of a lightweight ceramic Nano Glaze™ material.

Ask Yourself...

- Am I using safe cookware when I prepare my food?

- Are the bottom of my pots and pans all scratched, causing the material to lift?

- Am I using plastic in the microwave?

Your Wellness Strategies

- Check your cookware. Throw it out if it's health-hazardous.

- Buy glass containers to microwave and freeze your foods.

- Buy or order a new set of cookware.

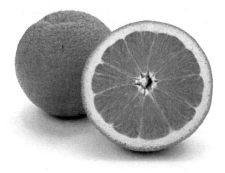

Chapter 45: Guilt Is Eating You Up!

– Andrée

*"If we are lucky, we can give in and rest without feeling guilty.
We can stop doing and concentrate on being."*
– Kathleen Norris

Like life, many movies have underlying messages that reflect what's right in front of us, if only we would listen intently and consciously.

In the movie "You've Got Mail", there is a scene where Meg Ryan gets into a cash-only checkout line at the grocery store – but has no cash on her. The cashier refuses to accept her credit card and the people in line behind her become cranky and tell her to use another line. Meg's character is embarrassed and keeps trying to convince the cashier to accept her credit card to avoid more of a scene. Then Tom Hanks appears to rescue her and pay her bill, but it only mortifies her further. She apologizes repeatedly and apparently feels very guilty about having to be rescued.

If we were often made to feel guilty as a child, we carry that learned guilt with us into adulthood. And believe it or not, if, as an adult we don't get a dose of guilt, we sometimes create a scenario to provoke it and get our fix. The consequence? We deprive ourselves of energy, focus, peace of mind, success and ultimately happiness – the price of guilt is high.

When do we feel guilty? Here are some scenarios that might sound familiar to you:

- Your mother calls and says, "You haven't called me in days!"
- Your significant other mentions that you haven't had sex in a while
- You see the pile of bills on your kitchen counter that are overdue
- You've been working long hours and you haven't spent much time with the kids
- You get a call from a charity looking for a donation but you say no because you can't afford to or you have already given to another charity

Guilt is a learned behavior that we develop as children. How can we say no and not feel guilty? First and foremost, it starts with knowing what we want, why we want it, and making sure others respect that.

Breaking Up with Guilt

The bottom line is that many of us give so much of ourselves because we're looking for approval. Approval-seeking behavior is an addictive behavior, as is the guilt we feel when we say no to other people's requests. This guilt is as much of an addiction as alcohol, drugs, food or sex. Guilt is incredibly powerful and has ruined lives.

Since guilt is a learned behavior, it is possible to unlearn it. But first we have to recognize that it's there. To unlearn guilt, ask yourself whether saying yes to everyone all of the time actually gets you more love and approval. To answer the question, no! The only thing it does is permit others to drive your life the way they want it to go with primary regard for themselves; and it leaves you exhausted. Isn't it ironic that the only person who doesn't make you feel guilty when you say no is yourself? Stop giving your life away; it's yours. Steer it the way you want it to go.

Ask Yourself...

- What is it costing you to say yes to everyone but yourself?

- What would you gain by getting back control of your own time?

- What is it costing you when you feel guilty?

- What would you gain by learning to accept your decisions and feel proud of them?

Your Wellness Strategies

- This week, pick one relationship where you know you need to take back control – e.g., a colleague who drags you out only to share her woes. Tell her you're busy. Tell her NO!

- Teach yourself how to feel good about your decisions by switching off your guilt. Simply ignore it – if you don't let it in, it'll stop knocking at your door.

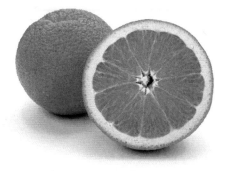

Chapter 46: What Is Wellness Chiropractic?

– Dr. Nathalie

"The doctor of the future will give no medicine, but will interest his patients in the care of the human frame, in diet, and in the cause and prevention of disease."

– Thomas Edison

The word 'chiropractic' comes from the Greek *chiros* and *praktikos,* meaning "done by hand". Chiropractic was founded in 1895 by D.D. Palmer, and it is now practiced in over 100 countries. Chiropractic is a safe and natural form of health care and is well-known for helping people with their aches and pains, but there is so much more to it than meets the eye!

Chiropractic care focuses on optimizing your body's own ability to function at its best. It achieves this by removing interference on the nervous system. Chiropractic care is a non-invasive and drug-free approach to health. Chiropractic does not include medications or prescription drugs, which often cover up important symptoms. A health symptom is your body's way of telling you that something is wrong and that it is an important signal one should not ignore. Medication may provide temporary relief but it often doesn't address the underlying issues. Chiropractic care focuses on addressing the cause of your symptoms as opposed to just camouflaging them. When your body is functioning properly, it has a tremendous ability to regulate and correct its own problems.

Subluxation

The spinal cord has 31 spinal nerves that exit between the spinal bones. Although the spinal column offers protection for these sensitive spinal nerves, their well-being can be disrupted if the spinal bones become misaligned. Subluxations are misalignments of the spine, incurred when the body is stressed beyond its capacity to adapt to its environment (physically, bio-chemically and psychologically). Subluxations create interference on the nervous system, which is the master system, and can compromise the vital communication between the brain and the rest of the body. Since we live our lives through our nervous system, we need to ensure that it is working at its best to achieve optimal health.

Sound confusing? Here is an analogy I tell my patients to help them really grasp the concept of a subluxation. What happens when you plug too many items in an electrical outlet? The breaker linked to this specific outlet will trip, right? If you go to the back panel and look at all the breakers, you will see that they are all aligned except one – the one you have tripped. A subluxation is just that – your body "tripping" because it has been stressed beyond its capacity to adapt. The stress could be a physical stress, a fall or hours in front of the computer. It could be a psychological stress, receiving bad news or an aggravating teenager. It could be a biochemical stress like eating greasy fast food or not drinking enough water. Do you see my point? Now, everybody has a different level at which they will "trip" their panel. We are all different depending on our body's capacity to adapt! My patients often think that there has to be a big physical event or activity to cause a spinal subluxation – not so! Subluxations can occur in any of the three dimensions – physical, psychological or biochemical.

Four Important Truths

Chiropractic is based on four self-evident truths:

1. The body is a self-healing, self-regulating organism.

    Self-healing – when you cut yourself you have the ability to heal because you are a living organism (this would not happen with a cadaver);

    Self-regulating – your heart is beating right now and you're not telling it to do so. Your stomach is also digesting the food you just ate without you commanding it to.

2. *"The nervous system is responsible for coordinating the function of every cell, tissue and organ in the body."* – <u>Gray's Anatomy</u>.

   This statement is rather self-explanatory – the nervous system is the master system and controls everything.

3. Subluxations (spinal misalignments) are the number one cause of interference with the body's innate ability to heal itself and self-regulate through the nervous system.

4. Chiropractic is the only healing science responsible for locating and correcting subluxations through the chiropractic adjustment, thereby restoring the body's ability to heal itself.

Types of Chiropractors

There are two types of chiropractors: a limited-scope chiropractor, who focuses mostly on pain relief, and a wellness chiropractor, who will deal not only with your body's signs and symptoms but will focus on the function of your nervous system and on the lifestyle stresses which may be causing your health challenges.

A wellness chiropractor will not only assess you for subluxations but also for the underlying causes in every dimensions of your life – physical, biochemical and psychological. A complete lifestyle evaluation will allow the chiropractor to make specific recommendations on those three dimensions and help diminish the negative stresses which may be perpetuating your subluxations. From time to time, you will be reassessed and your care program will be modified according to the changes and progress you have made in your life.

I always tell my patients that they have a choice in terms of what they want out of their chiropractic care. Symptomatic care may deal with a current health crisis, however wellness care will allow one to function optimally and effectively cope with lifestyle stresses. Studies are showing that patients under regular wellness care have better overall immune functions.

What is an Adjustment?

The method a chiropractor will use to correct a subluxation is called an adjustment. An adjustment involves a gentle and specific application of a force or touch to the spine in order to allow the body to restore normal spinal and nervous system functions. Several different techniques exist – they all have the same goal of removing the interference on one's nervous system.

Find a practitioner who uses a technique that works for you and that you are comfortable with.

You don't need to be in pain to see a chiropractor. Having a stress-free nervous system allows you to perform at your full potential. The longer you go with an unhealthy nervous system, the more devastating the effects are to your health and well-being. Often times, if we wait to have signs and symptoms, detrimental health consequences are already in progress. It's important to see a chiropractor who can maximize the efficiency of the nervous system by correcting subluxations for better health, longevity and quality of life.

Just as healthy eating, exercise and good rest are beneficial, chiropractic adjustments are crucial at all stages of life. This is a commitment to living your best life!

Athletes and high performers use chiropractic care to be and stay at the top of their games. An optimal nervous system can make the difference between first and second place in a race or a perfect golf swing. Examples of athletes using chiropractic care to perfect their performance are: Tiger Woods, Wayne Gretzky, Mary Lou Retton and Donovan Bailey.

Creating Wellness™ – Measuring Your Wellness Quotient

If you really want to know how "well" you are in all three dimensions we have talked about in this book, I suggest you book a wellness assessment at your local Creating Wellness™ Center.

Creating Wellness™ evaluations are fully integrated, doctor-led, customized wellness programs that focus on the three dimensions of your life. These assessments use breakthrough technology that scientifically measures, records and scores your level of wellness; physically, biochemically and emotionally. One of the unique features of the Creating Wellness™ System is the "Wellness Quotient." The Wellness Quotient is a score that rates your overall state of wellness – think of it as a Wellness IQ. It helps determine whether you're aging prematurely.

Based on your score, a specific three-dimensional customized wellness program will be created and customized to your unique needs. This will include a well-designed exercise program tailor-made for your performance goals and your level of physical fitness. It also includes a nutritional program customized to your specific caloric range, weight goals, and food preferences. Creating Wellness™ high quality supplements will respond to your unique biochemical requirements.

Another, and perhaps the most exciting and different component of the Creating Wellness™ plan, is the Wellness Coaching and Sound Advice programs. For the coaching portion, you meet on a weekly basis with a highly-trained, certified wellness coach who provides advice, tools and support to help you attain your health goals. For the Sound Advice portion, you receive a weekly custom-created audio segment filled with advice, solutions and powerful motivation in all three dimensions of your wellness. The Sound Advice program is designed by a team of chiropractors, physiologists, nutritionists, psychologists and health experts who cater to your unique needs and help you create the optimal wellness program that's right for you.

The Creating Wellness™ program can help you slow, stop, and even possibly reverse the aging process, and become an overall healthier person. To find out where the closest Creating Wellness™ Center is to you, visit www.creatingwellness.com.

ASK YOURSELF...

- Is my body sending me signals like headaches, back pain, fatigue or insomnia that I'm ignoring?
- Do I know if my body is working efficiently and optimally?
- Do I suspect that I may have subluxations affecting my health?
- Are my lifestyle stresses affecting my overall well-being?

YOUR WELLNESS STRATEGIES

- Schedule a wellness chiropractic assessment for you and your family.
- Identify and make positive changes to your lifestyle stressors.

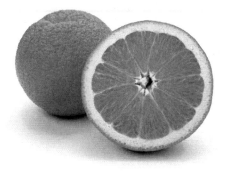

Chapter 47: The Coach And You!

– Andrée

Successful athletes, business people, health professionals, and the list goes on, use the services and expertise of coaches. Why? Well, they know that coaching is a process that can cause sustainable shifts in behavior. Through the coaching process, a coach assists the client in realizing their greatest potential necessary to live a spectacular life.

So how can coaching work for you? I think it's important to clarify that a coach is not a therapist. A coach is someone who truly believes in your potential and believes that you already have all the right answers residing inside of you. What a coach does is help you dig deep down inside to find these answers. A coach achieves this with you through questioning and exploring what you want most out of life.

A number of years ago when I was going through my own series of changes and transitions, I had the opportunity to attend a three-day intensive workshop that changed my life forever. Debbie Ford (www.debbieford. com) author of the book, The Dark Side of the Light Chasers and many other best-selling titles, lead a workshop which opened my eyes to the life of coaching. Throughout the workshop, I was surrounded by trained coaches who helped me decipher what changes I wanted to make in my life and what actions I needed to take to live a well-balanced life.

Since then, I have worked with certified coaches and achieved amazing results in my life, everything from developing healthy relationships to achieving a healthier body. I enjoyed the process so much I was certified in

2005 as an *Integrative Coach* through Debbie Ford's Integrative Coaching Institute.

So, think about it. Do you need to explore your needs and desires to make real and lasting changes? Do you need to find more balance in your life? Do you want to increase your earning potential or simply feel better in your body?

Through the use of questioning techniques, a coach can facilitate their client's own thought process to identify solutions and actions. A coach will support a client in setting appropriate goals and methods to assess their progress in relation to their goals. A coach will observe, listen, question and give feedback. They will also suggest creative tools and techniques to help you move forward toward your goals. These tools could include: training, reading material and various action plans.

Your coach becomes your accountability, a partner that ensures you are moving toward your goal. The coaching process is not meant to be a crutch to hang on to, but rather a process to empower you to take ownership and responsibility for your wellness – body, mind and soul.

A Life Coach!

A Life Coach, the type of coaching I provide, will help you integrate all the various areas of your life to achieve better balance. A coach will assist you in looking at the various parts of your life: health, relationships, finances, and environment. Over a period of months, a coach works with you to discover the best answers and best actions to achieve your goals.

Experience your best self, your best life. Be aware of who you are right now and who you want to be. Work with a coach. If you're looking for a coach in your area, check out the International Coaching Federation's website www.icf.org.

The coaching relationship assists you in staying focused on developing your *spectacular self*. This contributes to your talents, gifts and wisdom in your career, your relationship with yourself and others. It's all possible with the assistance of a coach.

Take a few minutes to visit my website www.synergieleadership.com for more information on coaching and on the services offered.

ASK YOURSELF...

- How could a coach help me find balance in my life?

- Where could I find the right type of coach for me?

- What would be the cost of not having a life or wellness coach?

YOUR WELLNESS STRATEGIES

- Write down in your journal the areas of your life you would like to discuss with a coach (i.e. your career, your health, your relationships).

- This week, visit www.synergieleadership.com to discover what coaching can do for you.

- This week, take time to talk to a coach and be receptive to the benefits of coaching.

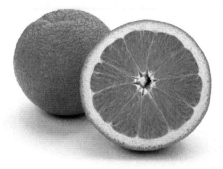

Chapter 48: Baby Steps

– Andrée

"In the book of life, the answers aren't in the back."
– Charlie Brown

Remember....baby steps!

In the beginning, there was confusion, denial, avoidance and, perhaps, even fear. Now here you are, armed and dangerous! In reading this book, you have acquired information, tips, tricks, knowledge on what wellness and balance is and what it means to you. At the end of each chapter, the "Ask Yourself..." portion guided you to create your own destination and ask important questions about your lifestyle and emotional well-being. The "Your Wellness Strategies" section made suggestions on how to create a road map to the healthy place where you want to be.

This book was meant to bring you awareness, so you can continue on your path to a healthier, more vibrant you and to live a spectacular life. Awareness was the first step, but it's just the beginning. While reading **Wellness on the Go**, you no doubt have made promises and commitments to yourself like changing your eating habits, your negative self-talk or reducing your stress. How will you ensure that you stay engaged? It takes *purpose, focus and enthusiasm* to hold on to what you want in life. You need those three ingredients to make it happen whether it's a fitter body, a better attitude or a completely new lifestyle. Take time to revisit your goals. What was your original intent when you bought this book? Was it simply to find out what wellness meant? Did you feel something missing in your life or did you feel the need to get fit and healthy?

Write down your *purpose*. Make it clear. Read it over and over again. Was it because you wanted to lose weight, or did you want to find out more about nutrition? Was it because you've been feeling a bit down about yourself and needed to boost your self-confidence or to stop feeling guilty for things? Once again, be clear about your purpose and the reason behind that purpose.

Next, keep your *focus*. You can achieve results by taking an action step every day toward your goal. It might be a very simple step like recording what you eat for lunch or making a commitment to go for a 20 minute walk everyday or doing a 10 minute meditation when you wake up. Whatever you choose to do, commit to it! Tell a friend about your commitment. Ask someone to keep you accountable. Remember this is for you and about you. You are the most important person in your life!

Enthusiasm is the best way to have fun with your plans. If you feel it's a chore or a task, in a short time, you will probably quit your new-found practice and forget about your goals. Create a fun reward for every little success along the way. Join a laughter yoga class, listen to your favorite comedian while walking – anything to make it fun. If you want to get fit, but you hate exercising, go dancing! Laugh a lot – laugh at yourself when you do it right and especially when you do it wrong. Or do as I did, buy a dog. The dog will get you walking at least three times per day and insist on playing outside.

Dr. Nathalie and I didn't want to leave you on your own for this journey. Our purpose was to accompany you on your path to a spectacular life. We have used our knowledge, research and life experience to help others.

Here is what we propose you do – the first baby step...

It takes 21 days to create a habit. What action can you take today and every day for the next 21 days to bring you closer to one of your goals?

YOUR WELLNESS STRATEGIES

- Find a coach. Uncover what area in your life needs the most attention and work jointly with your coach to develop new habits.

- Find a Wellness Chiropractor and/or a Creating Wellness™ Center with tools and technology to measure and monitor your level of wellness.

- Find natural health care practitioners who will help you achieve your wellness goals.

- Find an accountability partner. Travel in pairs on your road to success. It helps to have a co-pilot.

Slow down, take your time and make a commitment to yourself to make changes toward your wellness. And don't forget wellness is a journey, not a destination – enjoy the process and share it with your friends and family. Applaud yourself for taking time for you! We hope our book has raised your awareness about the different topics we discussed and restored your focus on what really matters – your **Wellness on the Go!**

References by Chapter

Chapter 1: Listen To Your Body, I Mean *Really* Listen!

Chiropractic Leadership Alliance. Conference notes & practitioner resources. Accessed 2006-2008 <www.subluxation.com>.

Creating Wellness™ Alliance. Conference notes & practitioner resources. Accessed 2006-2008 <www.creatingwellness.com>.

Hause, M. "Pain and the Nerve Root." Spine. 18.14 (1993): 2053.

Chapter 2: Awareness - Be Aware And Awake In Your Life

Maltz, Maxwell. The New Psycho-Cybernetics. Edited and Updated by Dan S. Kennedy and The Psycho-Cybernetics Foundation, Inc. New York: Prentice Hall Press, 2002.

Chapter 3: Wellness: What Does It Mean?

"Become an Optimist -- Live Longer". InteliHealth. 29 Aug. 2006. Aetna InteliHealth. Accessed 27 Aug. 2008 <www.intelihealth.com>.

Creating Wellness™ Alliance. Conference notes & practitioner resources. Accessed 2006-2008 <www.creatingwellness.com>.

Pilzer, Paul Zane. The Wellness Revolution. New York: John Wiley and Sons, 2002.

Selye, Hans. Stress Without Distress. New York: Lippencott, 1974.

Chapter 4: A Clear Purpose

Grabhorn, Lynn. Excuse Me, Your Life is Waiting. Charlottesville, VA: Hampton Roads Publishing Company, 2000.

Ford, Debbie. The Best Year of Your Life. New York: Harper Collins, 2005.

Losier, Michael J. Law of Attraction: The Science of Attracting More of What You Want and Less of What You Don't. Victoria, BC: Michael J. Losier, 2006.

Chapter 5: Protein, Carbs And Fat – What Am I Eating?

"Canola Quick Facts." Canola Council. 2007. Canola Council of Canada. 20 Nov. 2007 <http://www.canola-council.org>.

Church, T.S., C.E. Barlow, C.P. Earnest, J.B. Kampert, E.L. Priest, and S.N. Blair. "Associations between Cardiorespiratory Fitness and C-Reactive Protein in Men." Arteriosclerosis, Thrombosis, and Vascular Biology. 22.11 (1 Nov 2002): 1869-1876.

"Eat Well: The Protein Content of Common Foods." Healthy U: Your Pathway to Wellness. N.d. Northwestern Health Sciences University. Accessed 2008 <http://www.nwhealth.edu/healthyU/eatWell/protein3.html>.

Enig, Mary, Dr. and Sally Fallon. Eat Fat, Lose Fat: The Healthy Alternative to Trans Fats. New York: Penguin Group, 2006.

Gallop, Rick, and Emily Richards. Living the G.I Diet: Delicious Recipes and Real-Life Strategies to Lose Weight and Keep it Off. Toronto, ON: Random House Canada, 2003.

"Homocysteine, Folic Acid and Cardiovascular Disease." American Heart Association: Learn and Live. N.d. American Heart Association, Inc. Accessed 2008 <http://www.americanheart.org/presenter.jhtml?identifier=4677>.

"Inflammation, Heart Disease and Stroke: The Role of C-Reactive Protein." American Heart Association: Learn and Live. N.d. American Heart Association, Inc. Accessed 2008 <http://www.americanheart.org/presenter. jhtml?identifier=4648>.

Kim, Ben, Dr. "A Guide to Choosing Healthy Oils." Dr. Ben Kim: Experience Your Best Health. 10 Nov 2008. Dr. Ben Kim. Accessed 2008 <http://www. drbenkim.com/articles-oils.html>.

Mercola.com. Dr. Joseph Mercola. Accessed 2007-2008 <http://www.mercola.com>.

Mercola, Joseph, Dr. "Getting Tested for CRP May Save Your Life." Mercola. com. 26 Jan 2005. Dr. Joseph Mercola. Accessed 2008 <www.mercola.com>.

Mercola, Joseph, Dr., with Dr. Kendra Degen Pearsall. Take Control of Your Health. Schaumburg, IL: Dr. Joseph Mercola, 2007.

Mercola, Joseph, Dr. "Nutritional Typing™ Your Next Generation Key to Stupendous Lifelong Health (and Simpler Weight Management)" Mercola.com. Accessed 2007-2008 <http://products.mercola.com/nutritional-typing/>.

Nutrient Data Laboratory. "USDA National Nutrient Database for Standard Reference, Release 21." Agricultural Research Service. 2008. U.S. Department of Agriculture. Accessed 2008 <http://www.nal.usda.gov/fnic/foodcomp/search>.

Nutrient Value of Some Common Foods. Ottawa: Health Canada, 2008. E-booklet available at www.hc-sc.gc.ca. Accessed 2008 <http://www.hc-sc.gc.ca/fn-an/nutrition/fiche-nutri-data/nutrient_value-valeurs_nutritives-eng.php>.

Ogasawara, Sherry, Kyra Watter, Kerry Sherk, Linda Sampson, and Linda Hutton. Nutrition and Wellness Specialist Certification Manual, 2nd ed. Markham, ON: Can-Fit-Pro, July 2002.

Servan-Schreiber, David. Anticancer: A New Way of Life. Toronto, ON: Harper Collins, 2008.

Sizer, Frances, and Ellie Whitney. Nutrition Concepts and Controversies. 7th ed. Belmont, CA: Wadsworth Publishing Co., 1997.

Wolcott, William and Trish Fahey. The Metabolic Typing Diet. New York: Broadway Books, 2000.

Chapter 6: Learning To Read Food Labels

"Healthy Eating is in Store for You: Consumer Fact Sheets". Nutrition Labelling Education Centre. 2007. Canadian Diabetes Association and Dietitians of Canada. Accessed 2007-2008 <http://www.healthyeatingisinstore.ca>.

"Healthy Eating is in Store for You: FAQs". Nutrition Labelling Education Centre. 2005. Canadian Diabetes Association and Dietitians of Canada. Accessed 2007-2008 <http://www.healthyeatingisinstore.ca>.

Ogasawara, Sherry, Kyra Watter, Kerry Sherk, Linda Sampson, and Linda Hutton. Nutrition and Wellness Specialist Certification Manual, 2nd ed. Markham, ON: Can-Fit-Pro, July 2002.

Riley, Gay, M.S., R.D., C.C.N. "Before you Pig Out…" Men's Health. Oct. 2004: 142+.

Chapter 7: Processed Foods – What Exactly Are We Eating?

Dworkin, Andrea Sharon, and William Randall Kellas. Thriving in a Toxic World. Olivenhain, CA: Professional Preference, 1996.

Ebbeling, C.B., D.B. Pawlak, and D.S. Ludwig. "Childhood Obesity: Public Health Crisis, Common Sense Cure." The Lancet. 360.9331 (10 Aug. 2002): 473–482.

"E Number Index." UK Food Guide. 2007. Accessed 5 Mar. 2007 <http://www.ukfoodguide.net/enumeric.htm#antioxidants>.

"Food Additives May Affect Kids' Hyperactivity". WebMD. 24 May 2004. WebMD. Accessed 2007-2008 <http://www.webmd.com>.

Lambert, Craig. "The Way We Eat Now". Harvard Magazine. May-June 2004. Accessed 2007-2008 <http://www.harvardmagazine.com/on-line/050465.html>.

Mercola, Joseph, Dr. "How to Find Hidden MSG on Food Labels." Mercola.com. 2005. Dr. Joseph Mercola. Accessed 2007-2008 <www.mercola.com>.

Nutrition Action Healthletter. Toronto, ON: Centre for Science in the Public Interest, May 2008.

Schlosser Eric. Fast Food Nation: The Dark Side of the All-American Meal. New York: Houghton Mifflin, 2001.

Sizer, Frances, and Ellie Whitney. Nutrition Concepts and Controversies. 7th ed. Belmont, CA: Wadsworth Publishing Co., 1997.

"The Dyes Have It". Nutrition Action Healthletter. Toronto, ON: Centre for Science in the Public Interest, Oct. 2008.

Walker, M. et al. "Dietary Patterns and Risk of Prostate Cancer in Ontario, Canada". International Journal of Cancer. 10 Sep 2005; 116(4): 592-8.

Chapter 9: Less Is So Much More!

Ford, Debbie. The Dark Side of the Light Chasers: Reclaiming Your Power, Creativity, Brilliance, and Dreams. New York: Riverhead Books, 1998.

Ford, Debbie. "Integrative Coaching Certification Program." Course notes & resources. Institute for Integrative Coaching, San Diego, CA. Attended 2003-2005.

Chapter 10: Is It Worth Going Organic?

"10 Good Reasons to Go Organic." Organic Trade Association. N.d. Accessed 21 Dec. 2007 <http://www.ota.com/organic_and_you/10reasons.html?printable=1>.

Brady, Diane. "The Organic Myth." <u>Business Week</u>. 16 Oct. 2006. Accessed 21 Dec. 2007 <<u>http://www.businessweek.com/print/magazine/content/06_42/b4005001.htm?chan=g</u>>.

Canada. Canadian Food Inspection Agency. "Organic Products Regulations." Statutory Authority: Canada Agricultural Products Act. <u>Canada Gazette</u>. Vol. 140, No. 35 (2 Sep 2006). Accessed 2007-2008 <http://canadagazette. gc.ca/partI/2006/20060902/html/regle2-e.html>.

"Canada's New Government Certifies Organic Choice for Consumers." <u>Canadian Food Inspection Agency</u>. 21 July 2007. Accessed 2007-2008 <http://www.inspection.gc.ca/english/corpaffr/newcom/2007/20070721e. shtml>.

"Canadian National Organic Standard." <u>Whole Foods Market</u>. N.d. Accessed 19 July 2008 <http://www.wholefoodsmarket.com/issues/organic/standards_ canada.html>.

"Comprehensive Review of Pesticide Research Confirms Dangers: Family doctors highlight link between pesticide exposure and serious illnesses and disease; children particularly vulnerable." Toronto, ON: The Ontario College of Family Physicians, 23 Apr. 2004. <<u>www.ocfp.on.ca</u>>.

"Consumers Union Research Team Shows: Organic Foods Really DO Have Less Pesticides." <u>Consumers Union</u>. 8 May 2002. Accessed 23 Dec. 2007 <http://www.consumersunion.org/food/organicpr.htm>.

"The Full List: 43 Fruits and Veggies." <u>Environmental Working Group</u>. N.d. Accessed 2007 <http://www.ewg.org>.

Hansen, Nanette. "Organic Food Sales See Healthy Growth". 3 Dec 2004. <u>MSNBC</u>. Accessed 20 June 2006 <http://www.msnbc.msn.com/id/6638417/ >.

"List of Countries with Organic Agriculture Regulation." <u>Wikipedia</u>. Accessed 23 Dec. 2007 <http://en.wikipedia.org/wiki/List_of_countries_with_organic_ agriculture_regulation>.

Mercola, Joseph, Dr., with Rachael Droege. "How Do You Know if Your Food is Genetically Modified?" <u>Mercola.com</u>. 24 Jan. 2004. Dr. Joseph Mercola. Accessed 23 Dec. 2007. <http://www.mercola.com/display/PrintPage.aspx?do cid=28625&PrintPage=yes>

Mercola, Joseph, Dr., with Rachael Droege. "Why Do You Need Organic Food?" <u>Mercola.com</u>. 23 July 2003. Dr. Joseph Mercola. Accessed 21 Dec. 2007 <http://www.mercola.com/display/PrintPage.aspx?docid=27645&PrintPa ge=yes>.

"Organic Certification." <u>Wikipedia</u>. Accessed 23 Dec. 2007
<http://en.wikipedia.org/Organic_certification>.

"Organic Food." Wikipedia. Accessed 23 Dec. 2007 <http://en.wikipedia.org/
wiki/Organic_certification>.

"Organic Food Standards and Labels: The Facts". <u>National Organic Program</u>.
2006. USDA Agricultural Marketing Service. Accessed 6 June 2006
<http://www.ams.usda.gov>.

"Organics – Frequently Asked Questions." <u>Whole Foods Market</u>. 1 Aug. 2002.
Accessed 19 July 2008 <http://www.wholefoodsmarket.com/issues/organic/
faq.html>.

"Organic Labels." <u>Canadian Organic Growers</u>. 2006. Accessed 17 June 2008.
<http:/www.cog.ca/std_regs.htm>.

Schardt, David, with Lauren Clark. "Organic Food: Worth the Price?" <u>Nutrition
Action Healthletter</u>. Toronto, ON: Centre for Science in the Public Interest, July/
Aug. 2007.

Servan-Schreiber, David. <u>Anticancer: A New Way of Life</u>. Toronto, ON: Harper
Collins, 2008.

"Standards for Organic Agriculture." <u>Canadian General Standards Board</u>.
2006. Accessed 21 Dec. 2007 <http://www.tpsgc-pwgsc.gc.ca/cgsb/on_the_
net/organic/index-e.html>.

"Surprising Health Benefits of an Organic Diet." <u>Mercola.com</u>. 13 Apr. 2005.
Dr. Joseph Mercola. Accessed 23 Dec. 2007 <http://articles.mercola.com/
sites/articles/archive/2005/04/13/organic-diet.aspx>.

"Sustainability 101: The Benefits of Organics." <u>Home Grown Organic
Foods</u>. 2007. Accessed 21 Dec. 2007 <http:/www.hgof.ns.ca/index2.
php?function=ben_org>.

"Test Results: Full Data Set." <u>Shopper's Guide to Pesticides in Produce</u>. N.d.
E-book available at Food News. Environmental Working Group. Accessed
23 Dec. 2007 <http://www.foodnews.org/fulldataset.php>.

"When Buying Organic Pays (and Doesn't)." <u>Consumer Reports</u>. Feb. 2006.
Consumers Union. 21 Dec. 2007 <www.consumerreports.org>.

"When it Pays to Buy Organic." <u>Consumer Reports</u>. Feb. 2006. Consumers
Union. Accessed 21 Dec. 2007 <www.consumerreports.org>.

"Why Genetically Modified Crops Can Devastate Health." <u>Mercola.com</u>. 7 July 2003. Dr. Joseph Mercola. Accessed 23 Dec. 2007 <http://www.mercola.com/display/PrintPage.aspx?docid=27582&PrintPage=yes>.

Chapter 11: Do We Need MultiVitamins? Are They All Created Equal?

Aloisio, Ted. <u>Blood Never Lies</u>. Tamarac, FL: Llumina Press, 2004.

<u>Creating Wellness™ Alliance</u>. Conference notes & practitioner resources. Accessed 2006-2008 <www.creatingwellness.com>.

MacWilliam, Lyle. NutriSearch Comparative Guide to Nutritional Supplements. 4th ed. Vernon, BC: Northern Dimensions Publishing, 2007.

MacWilliam, Lyle. Nutritional Supplementation in Long Term Health (presentation). Chiropractic Leadership Summit 2007. Chiropractic Leadership Alliance. Indian Lakes Resort, Bloomingdale, IL. 5-6 Oct. 2007.

Mercola, Joseph, Dr. "Your Multivitamin May Not be All It Claims to Be" <u>Mercola.com</u>. Dr. Joseph Mercola. Accessed 2007-2008 <http://articles.mercola.com/whole-foods-multivitamin>.

Chapter 12: The Power Of Omega-3

Bibus, Douglas M., et al. "Bioavailability Studies of Emulsified Flavored Fish Oil." The University of Minnesota, Austin, MN. 21 Jan. 2000.

Connor, William E., "Importance of n-3 Fatty Acids in Health and Disease." American Journal of Clinical Nutrition. 71.1 (Jan. 2000): 171S-175S. American Society for Clinical Nutrition. Accessed 17 Feb. 2008 <http://www.ajcn.org/cgi>.

<u>Douglas Laboratories</u>. Accessed 2007-2008 <<u>www.douglaslabs.com</u>>.

"Fish Oil Benefits/ Clinical Studies." <u>XTend-Life Natural Products</u>. Accessed 1 Sep. 2007 <www.truthaboutomega3.com/benefit.html>.

Holub, B.J., Dr. "Clinical nutrition: 4. Omega-3 Fatty Acids in Cardiovascular Care." <u>CMAJ</u>. 166.5 (5 Mar. 2002). Canadian Medical Association. Accessed 17 Feb. 2008 <http://www.cmaj.ca>.

Holub, B.J., Dr. "Fish Oils and Cardiovascular Disease." <u>CMAJ</u>. 141.10 (15 Nov. 1989): 1063.

Larsen, Hans R. "Fish Oils: The Essential Nutrients." <u>International Health News</u>. Issue 103 (July 2000). Accessed 2007-2008 <www.vvv.com/HealthNews/fish_oils.htm>.

Liebman, Bonnie. "Omega Medicine? Is Fish Oil Good for What Ails You?" Nutrition Action Healthletter. Toronto, ON: Centre for Science in the Public Interest, Oct. 2007.

MacWilliam, Lyle. NutriSearch Comparative Guide to Nutritional Supplements. 4th ed. Vernon, BC: Northern Dimensions Publishing, 2007.

Mercola, Joseph, Dr., with Rachael Droege. "What You Must Know Before You Eat Fish." Mercola.com. 9 Aug. 2003. Dr. Joseph Mercola. Accessed 17 June 2008 <http://articles.mercola.com/sites/articles/archive/2003/08/09/fish-mercury-part-one.aspx>.

Metagenics. Accessed 2007-2008 <www.metagenics.com>.

Poliquin, Charles, and Dr. Mark Houston. "Fishing for Supplements: Thirteen Reasons to Use Fish Oils to Get Lean." Poliquin. Accessed 1 Sep. 2007 <www.charlespoliquin.com>.

Saynor, R. and T. Gillott. "Changes in Blood Lipids and Fibrinogen with a Note on Safety in a Long Term Study on the Effects of n-3 Fatty Acids in Subjects Receiving Fish Oil Supplements and Followed for Seven Years." Lipids. Vol. 27 (July 1992): 533-38.

Sizer, Frances, and Ellie Whitney. Nutrition Concepts and Controversies. 7th ed. Belmont, CA: Wadsworth Publishing Co., 1997.

Chapter 13: Looking At Stress Creatively

Kabat-Zinn, Jon. Wherever You Go, There You Are: Mindfulness Meditation in Everyday Life. New York: Hyperion, 1994.

Posen, David B., M.D. The Little Book of Stress Relief. Toronto, ON: Key Porter Books, 2003.

Selye, Hans. Stress without Distress. New York: Signet, 1975.

"Stress (Biological)." Wikipedia. Accessed 2007-2008 <http://en.wikipedia.org/wiki/Stress_(medicine)>.

Chapter 14: Deodorant – Sometimes The Facts Stink

"Antiperspirant/ Deodorant Scores." Skin Deep: Cosmetic Safety Database. Environmental Working Group. Accessed 2008 <http://www.cosmeticsdatabase.com>.

"Concern over Deodorants and Breast Cancer." Mercola.com. 28 Jan. 2004. Dr. Joseph Mercola. Accessed 2007-2008 <http://articles.mercola.com/sites/articles/archive/2004/01/28/deodorant-cancer.aspx>.

Darbre, P.D. "Aluminium, Antiperspirants and Breast Cancer." Journal of Inorganic Biochemistry. 99.9: (Sep. 2005): 1912-1919.

Darbre, P.D. "Underarm Cosmetics and Breast Cancer." Journal of Applied Toxicology. 23.2 (Mar./Apr. 2003): 89-95.

Huber, Colleen, Dr. "Cause for Concern: Carcinogens in Bath Products." Mercola.com. 2007. Dr. Joseph Mercola. Accessed 2007-2008 <www.mercola.com>.

McGrath, K.G. "An Earlier Age of Breast Cancer Diagnosis Related to More Frequent Use of Antiperspirants/Deodorants and Underarm Shaving." European Journal of Cancer Prevention. 12.6 (Dec. 2006): 479-85.

Smith, Elizabeth, M.D. "Xenoestrogen: The Cause of Fibrocystic Breast Disease – How to Avoid Xenoestrogens." Fibrocystic Breast Disease. Accessed 4 Mar. 2007 <http:/www.fibrocystic.com/xeno.htm>.

Chapter 15: Breathe Clean

"Air Cleaning Devices." American Lung Association. Accessed 18 Mar. 2008 <http://www.lungusa.org/site/apps/s/content.asp?c=dvLUK9O0E&b=3569>.

"Air Cleaning Devices for the Home: Frequently Asked Questions." Air Resources Board. 4 Feb. 2005. California Environmental Protection Agency. Accessed 18 Mar. 2008. <www.arb.ca.gov/research/indoor/aircleaner.htm>.

"Air Purifier Ratings." Consumer Reports. November 2007. Consumers Union. Accessed 18 Mar. 2008. <http://www.consumerreports.org/cro/appliances/air-cleaners-1005/overview/index.htm>.

"ARB Warns – Danger from Popular "Air Purifying" Machines." California Air Resources Board. 20 Jan. 2005. California Environmental Protection Agency. Accessed 18 Mar. 2008. <http://www.arb.ca.gov/newsrel/nr012005.htm>.

Brooks, Bradford O., Gary M. Utter, James A. DeBroy, and Roger D. Schimke. "Indoor Air Pollution: An Edifice Complex." Journal of Toxicology: Clinical Toxicology. 29.3 (1991): 315-374.

"Health Canada Warns the Public About Air Cleaners Designed to Intentionally Generate Ozone." Health Canada. 13 Apr. 1999. Accessed 2007-2008 <http://www.hc-sc.gc.ca/english/protection/warnings/1999/99_62e.html>.

"Health Update: Indoor Ozone Generators Sold As Air Purifiers." Presentation at the ARB Board Meeting. 20 Jan. 2005. California Air Resources Board, California Environmental Protection Agency. Accessed 18 Mar. 2008 <http://www.arb.ca.gov/research/indoor/ozone.htm>.

Mercola.com. Dr. Joseph Mercola. Accessed 2007-2008 <www.mercola. com>.

National Air Filtration Association. Accessed 18 Mar. 2008 <www.nafahq.org>.

Oliver L.C., and B.W. Shackleton. "The Indoor Air We Breathe." Indoor Air Quality: Public Health Report. 113.5 (1998): 398-409.

"Ozone Generators That Are Sold as Air Cleaners: An Assessment of Effectiveness and Health Consequences." U.S. Environmental Protection Agency: Indoor Air Quality (IAQ). 26 July 2004. Accessed 2007-2008 <http://www.epa.gov/iaq/pubs/ozonegen.html>.

Power5 Pro. Product Information Sheet. Irvine, CA: Nikken Inc., 2008.

"Reducing your Exposure to Particulate Pollutants: Fact Sheet." Air Resources Board. Dec. 2001. California Environmental Protection Agency. Accessed 18 Mar. 2008 <http://www.arb.ca.gov/research/indoor/pmfactsheet.pdf>.

Chapter 16: Just Breathe

Latulippe, Lise. Owner of Adi Shakti Yoga Centre, Orleans, Ontario. Personal interviews & informational verification. 2007-2008 <http://www.adishaktiyogacentre.com>.

Lewis, Dennis. The Tao of Natural Breathing: For Health, Well-Being, and Inner Growth. Berkeley, CA: Rodmell Press: 2006.

Chapter 17: Adjusting Your Inner PH For Optimal Health

Aloisio, Ted. Blood Never Lies. Tamarac, FL: Llumina Press, 2004.

"Approximate pH of Foods and Food Products." U.S. Food and Drug Administration: Center for Food Safety and Applied Nutrition. April 2007. U.S. Department of Health and Human Services. Accessed 24 Sep. 2008. <http://www.cfsan.fda.gov/~comm/lacf-phs.html>.

"Balancing Acid/Alkaline Foods." Trans4Mind. Accessed 15 June 2008 <http://www.trans4mind.com/nutrition/pH.html>.

Baroody, Theodore A, Jr. Alkalize or Die. 8th ed. Waynesville, NC: Holographic Health Press, 1991.

Genuine Health. Accessed 2007-2008 <www.genuinehealth.com>.

Karp, Gerald. Cell and Molecular Biology. 4th ed. Hoboken, NJ: John Wiley & Sons, 2005.

"List of Alkaline Foods." <u>Energise for Life</u>. 2005. Accessed 2007-2008 <http://www.energiseforlife.com/list_of_alkaline_foods.php>.

Marieb, Elaine N. <u>Human Anatomy & Physiology</u>. 5th ed. San Francisco, CA: Benjamin Cummings, 2001.

Young, Robert, Ph.D., with Shelley Redford Young. <u>The pH Miracle: Balance your Diet, Reclaim your Health</u>. New York: Warner Books, Inc., 2002.

Chapter 18: Benefits Of Greens

Ben-Arye, E., E. Goldin, D. Wengrower, A Stamper, R Kohn, and E Berry. "Wheat Grass Juice in the Treatment of Active Distal Ulcerative Colitis: A Randomized Double-Blind Placebo-Controlled Trial." <u>Scandinavian Journal of Gastroenterology</u>. Norway: Informa Healthcare, April 2002. 37.4: 444-9.

"Chlorella – A Natural Wonder Supplement." <u>Mercola.com.</u> N.d. Dr. Joseph Mercola. Accessed 11 April 2007 <www.mercola.com>.

'Chlorophyll.' <u>Alternative Healthzine.</u> 2005. Accessed 2007-2008 <www.alternative-healthzine.com/html/0500_2.html>.

"Chlorophyll: Definition, Chlorophyll Health Benefits, Photosynthesis and Other Uses." <u>Dietary Fiber Food.</u> 30 Aug. 2007. Accessed 2007-2008 <www.dietaryfiberfood.com/chlorophyll.php>.

<u>Genuine Health</u>. Accessed 2007-2008 <www.genuinehealth.com>.

Meyerowitz, Steve. <u>Wheatgrass: Nature's Finest Medicine: The Complete Guide to Using Grass Foods & Juices to Revitalize Your Health</u>, 6th ed., Summertown,
TN: Book Publishing Company, 1999.

<u>Nikken</u>. Accessed 2008 <www.nikken.com>.

Chapter 19: Measure Up!

"BMI Classification." <u>WHO: World Health Organization</u>. 2006. United Nations. Accessed 2007-2008 <http://www.who.int/bmi/index.jsp?introPage=intro_3.html>.

"Body Fat Analyzer – the FUTREX 6100." <u>Creating Wellness™ Alliance</u>. Information for centres. Accessed 2007-2008 <www.creatingwellness.com>.

"Body Mass Index Table." <u>National Heart Lung and Blood Institute</u>. N.d. National Institutes of Health. Accessed 2007-2008 <http://www.nhlbi.nih.gov/guidelines/obesity/bmi_tbl.htm>.

Gallagher, Dympna, Steven B Heymsfield, Moonseong Heo, Susan A Jebb, Peter R Murgatroyd and Yoichi Sakamoto. "Healthy Percentage Body Fat Ranges: An Approach for Developing Guidelines Based on Body Mass Index." American Journal of Clinical Nutrition. 72. 3 (Sep 2000): 694-701.

Ogasawara, Sherry, Kyra Watter, Kerry Sherk, Linda Sampson, and Linda Hutton. Nutrition and Wellness Specialist Certification Manual, 2nd ed. Markham, ON: Can-Fit-Pro, July 2002.

"Waist to Hip Ratio". Access 2007-2008 <http://www.topendsports.com/testing/tests/WHR.htm>.

Chapter 20: The Little Voice Inside Your Head

Laroche, Loretta. Life Is Short – Wear Your Party Pants [Audiobook]. Carlsbad, CA: Hay House, 2003.

Laroche, Loretta. The Joy of Stress with Loretta Laroche: How to Prevent Hardening of the Attitude. Producer Laurie Donnelly. WGBH Boston in association with The Humor Potential Inc. 1995. DVD. WGBH Educational Foundation, 2002.

Maltz, Maxwell. The New Psycho-Cybernetics. Edited and Updated by Dan S. Kennedy and The Psycho-Cybernetics Foundation, Inc. New York: Prentice Hall Press, 2002.

Chapter 21: Cardiovascular Training – The Heart Of The Matter

ACSM's Guidelines for Exercise Testing and Prescription. 7th ed. Baltimore, MD: Lipincott Williams & Wilkins, 2005.

Hutton, Janice. Personal Trainer Specialist Manual. 3rd ed. Markham, ON: Can-Fit-Pro, Mar. 2006.

McArdle, W.D., F.I. Katch, and V.L. Katch. Sports and Exercise Nutrition. New York, NY: Lippincott Williams & Wilkins, 1999.

Mercola.com. Dr. Joseph Mercola. Accessed 2007-2008 <www.mercola.com>.

Pollock M.L., G.A. Gaesser, and J.D. Butcher, et al. "ACSM Position Stand: The Recommended Quantity and Quality of Exercise for Developing and Maintaining Cardio-respiratory and Muscular Fitness and Flexibility in Healthy Adults." Medicine & Science in Sports & Exercise. 30.6 (June 1998): 975-978.

Sears, Al, M.D. PACE: Rediscover Your Native Fitness. Wellington, FL: Wellness Research & Consulting Inc., 2006.

Chapter 22: Strength Training – "Tour De Force"

Bayer J. "Free Weights versus Machines." Fox Sports. 2007. Microsoft. Accessed 2007-2008 <http://msn.foxsports.com>.

Hutton, Janice. Personal Trainer Specialist Manual. 3rd ed. Markham, ON: Can-Fit-Pro, Mar. 2006.

Seguin Rebecca, and Miriam E. Nelson. "The Benefits of Strength Training for Older Adults." American Journal of Preventive Medicine. 25.3.Suppl.2 (Oct. 2003): 144-149.

Vehrs, Pat R., Ph.D. "Strength Training in Children and Teens: Dispelling Misconceptions – Part One." ACSM's Health and Fitness Journal. 9.4 (July/Aug. 2005): 8-12.

"Weight Training Guidelines: American College of Sports Medicine Recommendations and Position Stance. (ACSM 1995)." Summarized on ExRx. net. Accessed 2007-2008 <www.exrx.net/WeightTraining/Guidelines.html>.

Chapter 24: Yoga For Your Body, Mind And Soul

"Getting Started – Beginner's Guide to Yoga." A-B-C of Yoga. Accessed 2007-2008 <http://www.abc-of-yoga.com/yogabeginnersguide.asp>.

Latulippe, Lise. Owner of Adi Shakti Yoga Centre, Orleans, Ontario. Personal interviews & informational verification. 2007-2008 <http://www.adishaktiyogacentre.com>.

Yoga Holidays and Retreats. Accessed 2007-2008 <www.yogaholidays.net>.

Chapter 25: Boning Up

Bharadwaj S., A.G.T. Naidu, G.V. Betageri, N.V. Prasadarao, and A.S. Naidu. "Milk Ribonuclease-Enriched Lactoferrin Induces Positive Effects on Bone Turnover Markers in Postmenopausal Women." Osteoporosis International. Online First (27 Jan 2009): published online.

Bio-replenishment: OsteoDenx. Brochure. Irvine, CA: Nikken Inc., 2007. <http://www.nikken.com>.

"Calcium and Strong Bones." Physicians Committee for Responsible Medicine (PCRM). 2001. Accessed 2007-2008 <http://www.pcrm.org/health/prevmed/strong_bones.html>.

"Don't Drink Your Milk!" Mercola.com. N.d. Dr. Joseph Mercola. Accessed 2007-2008 <http://www.mercola.com/article/milk/no_milk.htm>.

"Do You Really Need Calcium to Build Strong Bones?" Mercola.com. 7 June 2003. Dr. Joseph Mercola. Accessed 2007-2008 <http://articles.mercola.com/sites/articles/archive/2003/06/07/calcium-bones.aspx>.

Graci, Sam, Carolyn Demarco and Leticia Rao. The Bone Building Solution. Missisauga, ON: John Wiley & Sons Canada, 2006.

Grant, William B. "Reduce Your Risk of Cancer with Sunlight Exposure." Mercola.com. 31 Mar. 2004. Dr. Joseph Mercola. Accessed 2007-2008 <http://articles.mercola.com/sites/articles/archive/2004/03/31/cancer-sunlight.aspx>.

Murphree, Rodger H., II. "Osteopenia, Osteoporosis and Osteonecrosis". NutriNews (Bone Health). Nov. 2007. Douglas Laboratories. Accessed 2007-2008 <http://www.douglaslabs.com/listpdfs.cfm?cat=nutrinews>.

Prince, Richard L., Amanda Devine, Satvinder S. Dhaliwal, and Ian M. Dick. "Effects of Calcium Supplementation on Clinical Fracture and Bone Structure." Archives of Internal Medicine. 166.8 (24 Apr. 2006): 869-875.

Rosenberg, Martha. "Will Fosamax be the New Vioxx?" medHeadlines. 26 Jan 2009. Synapse Medical Publishers, Inc. Accessed 30 Jan 2009 <http://medheadlines.com/2009/01/26/will-fosamax-be-the-new-vioxx>.

Chapter 26: Vitamin D, Sunshine And Sunscreen

Agar, N.S., Halliday G.M., Barnetson R.StC., Ananthaswamy H.N., Wheeler M., and Jones A.M. "The Basal Layer in Human Squamous Tumors Harbors More UVA than UVB Fingerprint Mutations: A Role for UVA in Human Skin Carcinogenesis." Proceedings of the National Academy of Sciences of the USA (PNAS). 101.14 (6 Apr. 2004): 4954-9.

Bestak, R., R. StC. Barnetson, M.R. Nearn, and G.M. Halliday. "Sunscreen Protection of Contact Hypersensitivity Responses from Chronic Solar-Simulated Ultraviolet Irradiation Correlates with the Absorption Spectrum of the Sunscreen." Journal of Investigative Dermatology. 105.3 (Sep. 1995): 345-51.

Diffey, Brian L. "What is Light?" Photodermatology, Photoimmunology &Photomedicine. 18.2 (9 May 2002): 68-74.

Grant, William B. "An Estimate of Premature Cancer Mortality in the U.S. Due to Inadequate Doses of Solar Ultraviolet-B Radiation." Cancer. 94.6 (15 Mar. 2002): 1867-75.

Grant, William B. "Reduce Your Risk of Cancer with Sunlight Exposure." Mercola.com. 31 Mar. 2004. Dr. Joseph Mercola. Accessed 2007-2008 <http://articles.mercola.com/sites/articles/archive/2004/03/31/cancer-sunlight.aspx>.

Haywood R., P. Wardman, R. Sanders, and C. Linge. "Sunscreens Inadequately Protect Against Ultraviolet-A-Induced Free Radicals in Skin: Implications for Skin Aging and Melanoma?" Journal of Investigative Dermatology. 121.4 (Oct. 2003): 862-8.

Mercola, Joseph, Dr., with Rachael Droege. "Trash Your Sunscreen and Other Summer Sun Tips." Mercola.com. 26 May 2004. Dr. Joseph Mercola. Accessed 9 Dec. 2007 <http://articles.mercola.com/sites/articles/archive/2004/05/26/summer-sun.aspx>.

Patagonia. Accessed 2007-2008 <www.patagonia.com>.

"Skin Cancer Facts." The Skin Cancer Foundation. 2007. Accessed 20 Mar 2007 <http://www.skincancer.org/skincancer_facts.php>.

"Skin Safety 101." Skin Deep: Cosmetic Safety Database. N.d. Environmental Working Group. Accessed 2008 <http://www.cosmeticsdatabase.com/special/sunscreens2008/report_skinsafety.php>.

Standley, Vincent. "Which Sunscreen Should I Choose?" The Green Guide. 14 June 2005. National Geographic. Accessed 2008 <http:/thegreenguide.com/doc/ask/sunblock>.

"Sunscreen Summary: What Works & What's Safe." Skin Deep: Cosmetic Safety Database. N.d. Environmental Working Group. Accessed 2008 <http://www.cosmeticsdatabase.com/special/sunscreens2008/summary.php>.

"Sunscreens: Sunscreen Home." Skin Deep: Cosmetic Safety Database. N.d. Environmental Working Group. Accessed 2008 <www.cosmeticsdatabase.com/sunscreens>.

Vasil, Adria. "The Dark Side of Sunscreen Chemicals." Ewg.org (re-posted from Torontonow.com). 27 June 2007. Environmental Working Group. Accessed 2008 <http://www.ewg.org/node/21938>.

"Who's Protecting Us?" Skin Deep: Cosmetic Safety Database. N.d. Environmental Working Group. Accessed 2008 <http://www.cosmeticsdatabase.com/special/sunscreens2008/report_protection.php>.

Chapter 27: Laughter Is The Sunshine Of Your Life

Laroche, Loretta. Life Is Short – Wear Your Party Pants [Audiobook]. Carlsbad, CA: Hay House, 2003.

Laroche, Loretta. The Joy of Stress with Loretta Laroche: How to Prevent Hardening of the Attitude. Producer Laurie Donnelly. WGBH Boston in association with The Humor Potential Inc. 1995. DVD. WGBH Educational Foundation, 2002.

"Laughter." Wikipedia. Accessed 2007-2008 <http://en.wikipedia.org/wiki/Laughter>.

Laughter.com. 1 Apr. 1998. Sharon Braverman. Accessed 2007-2008 <http://www.laughter.com>.

Scott, Elizabeth, M.S. "Stress Management and the Health Benefits of Laughter." About.com. 22 Apr. 2008. The New York Times Company. Accessed 2008 <http://stress.about.com/od/stresshealth/a/laughter.htm>.

Chapter 28: "Whey" To Go!

Bertheau, Cynthia, ed. "Whey Proteins and Body Composition." U.S. Dairy Export Council. 2004. Accessed 25 Dec. 2007 <http://usdec.files.cms-plus.com/Publications/WheyBodyComposition_English.pdf>.

Bounous, G. "Whey Protein Concentrate (WPC) and Glutathione Modulation in Cancer Treatment." Anticancer Research. 20.6c (2000): 4785-92.

Bouthegourd, J-C.J., S.M. Roseau, L. Makarios-Lahham, P.M. Leruyet, D.G. Tomé, and P.C. Even. "A Preexercise (X-Lactalbumin-Enriched Whey Protein Meal Preserves Lipid Oxidation and Decrease Adiposity in Rats." American Journal of Physiology – Endocrinology and Metabolism. 283.3 (Sep. 2002): E65-E572.

Brink, Will. Brink's Body Building Revealed. Internet Publications Group, 2007. E-book available at Brinkzone.com. Accessed 25 Dec 2007 <www.brinkzone.com>.

Doherty, Timothy J. "Invited Review: Aging and Sarcopenia." Journal of Applied Physiology. 95.4 (Oct. 2003): 1717-1727.

Mercola.com. Dr. Joseph Mercola. Accessed 2007-2008 <www.mercola.com>.

Rennie, Michael J., and Kevin D. Tipton. "Protein and Amino Acid Metabolism During and After Exercise and the Effects of Nutrition." Annual Review of Nutrition. 20 (July 2000): 457-483.

Servan-Schreiber, David. Anticancer: A New Way of Life. Toronto, ON: Harper Collins, 2008.

"Whey Protein FAQ's." Whey Protein Institute. Accessed 25 Dec. 2007 <http://www.wheyoflife.org/faq.cfm>.

Chapter 29: The Soy Controversy

"Benefits of Soy Products." Soy Info Online! 2007. Accessed 1 Sep. 2007 <http://www.soyinfo.com/benefits.shtml>.

Brink, Will. Brink's Body Building Revealed. Internet Publications Group, 2007. E-book available at Brinkzone.com. Accessed 25 Dec 2007 <www.brinkzone.com>.

Constantinou, A. "Interaction Between Genistein and Estrogen Receptors May Enhance Mammary Tumor Growth." American Association for Cancer Research. April 2000. reported in Guterman, L. "The Power of Soy." Today's Chemist at Work (publication of the American Chemical Society). June 2000.

Daniel, Kaayla T., PhD. The Whole Soy Story: The Dark Side of America's Favorite "Health Food". Winona Lake, IN: New Trends Publishing: 2007.

Dees, C., J.S. Foster, S. Ahamed, and J. Wimalasena. "Dietary Estrogens Stimulate Human Breast Cells to Enter the Cell Cycle." Environmental Health Perspectives. Vol.105, Suppl.3 (Apr. 1997): 633-6.

Divi, R.L., H.C. Chang, and D.R. Doerge. "Anti-Thyroid Isoflavones from Soybean." Biochemical Pharmacology. 54.10 (15 Nov. 1997): 1087-96.

Fallon, Sally, Mary G. Enig. "Cinderella's Dark Side." Mercola.com. 9 Apr. 2000. Dr. Joseph Mercola. Accessed 2007-2008 <http://articles.mercola.com/sites/articles/archive/2000/04/09/soy-research-update.aspx>.

Gurd, Vreni. "The Soy Controversy." Wellness Tips. 2 Apr. 2006. Accessed 2007-2008 <http://home.ezezine.com/221/221-2006.04.02.08.00.archive.html>.

Hilakivi-Clarke, L., et al, "Maternal Exposure to Genistein during Pregnancy Increases Carcinogenic-Induced Mammary Tumorigenisis in Female Rat Offspring." The Oncology Report. Vol. 6 (Sep.-Oct. 1999): 1089-95.

Katsuyama, H., S. Ideguchi, et al. "Usual Dietary Intake of Fermented Soybeans (Natto) is Associated with Bone Mineral Density in Pre-Menopausal Women." Journal of Nutritional Science and Vitaminology (Tokyo). 48.3 (2002): 207-215.

Kotsopoulos, D., F.S. Dalais, Y.-L. Liang, B.P. McGrath, H.J. Teede. "The Effects of Soy Protein Containing Phytoestrogen on Menopausal Symptoms in Post-menopausal Women." Climacteric – The Journal of the International Menopause Society. 3.3 (Sep. 2000): 161-167.

Liener, I. E. "Hemagglutinins in Foods." Chapter 6 in Toxicants <u>Occurring Naturally in Foods</u>. Washington, D.C.: National Academy of Sciences/National Research Council, 1966. Publication 1354: pp. 51-7.

Mercola, Joseph, Dr. "Think Soy is Healthy? Here's Why It's Not As Good As You Think." <u>Mercola.com</u>. 21 Apr. 2004. Dr. Joseph Mercola. Accessed 2007-2008 <http://articles.mercola.com/sites/articles/archive/2004/04/21/soy-health.aspx>.

Murkies A.L., G. Wilcox, and S.R. Davis. "Clinical Review 92: Phytoestrogens." <u>American Journal of Physiology – Endocrinology and Metabolism</u>. 83.2 (Feb. 1998): 297-303.

"Myths and Truths about Soy Foods." <u>Soy Online Services.</u> 2007. Soy Information Service. Accessed 26 Dec. 2007 <http://www.soyonlineservice.co.nz/03soymyths.htm>.

Petrakis, N. L., et al, "Stimulatory Influence of Soy Protein Isolate on Breast Secretion in Pre- and Post-Menopausal Women." <u>Cancer Epidemiology and Biological Previews</u>. Vol. 5 (1996): 785-94.

"Powerful Benefits of Soy." <u>HealthCastle.com</u>. Feb. 2006. Healthcastle Nutrition, Inc. Accessed 1 Sep. 2007 <<u>www.healthcastle.com/herb_soy.shtml</u>>.

Shurtleff, William, and Akiko Aoyagi. "Protein Quality (NPU) of Various Foods [Fig. 2.3]." <u>The Book of Tempeh</u>. 2nd ed. Berkeley, CA: Ten Speed Press, Sep. 2001. pp. 31.

"Soy - One of the Nine Most Common Food Allergens." <u>Health Canada</u>. 20 Apr. 2004. Accessed 2007-2008 <<u>http://www.hc-sc.gc.ca/fn-an/securit/allerg/fa-aa/allergen_soy-soja_e.html</u>>.

Stob, M. "Estrogens in Foods." Chapter 2 in <u>Toxicants Occurring Naturally in Foods</u>. Washington, D.C.: National Academy of Sciences/National Research Council, 1966. Publication 1354: pp. 18-23.

Terrain, Mary Vance. "The Dark Side of Soy: Is America's Favorite Health Food Making Us Sick?" <u>Utne Reader</u>. July/Aug. 2007. Ogden Publications, Inc. Accessed 2007-2008 <http://www.utne.com/2007-07-01/Science-Technology/The-Dark-Side-of-Soy.aspx>.

Torum, B. "Nutritional Quality of Soybean Protein Isolates Studies in Children of Preschool Age." <u>Soy Protein and Human Nutrition</u>. Harold L. Wicke, et al, eds. New York: Academic Press, 1979.

Chapter 30: Gluten – Are You Sensitive To It?

Case, Shelly. Gluten-Free Diet: A Comprehensive Resource Guide. Regina, SK: Case Nutrition Consulting, 2006.

Fasano A, Berti I, Gerarduzzi T, et al. Prevalence of celiac disease in at-risk and not-at-risk groups in the United States. Archives of Internal Medicine. 2003;163(3):268-292.

"Following a Gluten-Free Diet." Beth Israel Deaconess Medical Center (A Teaching Hospital of Harvard Medical School). Jan. 2006. Accessed 2007-2008 <http://www.bidmc.harvard.edu>.

GlutenFree.com. Accessed 2007-2008 <http://www.glutenfree.com>.

"Gluten-Free Diet." Wikipedia. Accessed 2007-2008 <http://en.wikipedia.org/wiki/Gluten-free_diet>.

Huntington, Anna Seaton. "A Debilitating Disease That Is Often Unknown." NYTimes.com. 9 Oct. 2008. The New York Times. Accessed 2008 <http://www.nytimes.com/2008/10/10/sports/othersports/10celiac.html>.

"Organic Coconut Flour." Tropical Traditions. Accessed 2007-2008 <http://www.tropicaltraditions.com/organic_coconut_flour.htm>.

Chapter 32: Water And Your Body

Alive.com (website for Alive magazine). 2005. Alive Publishing Group. Accessed 2007-2008 <http://www.alive.com>.

Aloisio, Ted. Blood Never Lies. Tamarac, FL: Llumina Press, 2004.

Batmanghelidj, F., M.D. The Water Cure. Global Health Solutions, Inc. Accessed 29 May 2007 <www.watercure.com>.

Batmanghelidj, F., M.D. Your Body's Many Cries for Water. Vienna, VA: Global Health Solutiuons, 1997.

Bragg, Patricia, and Paul C. Bragg, M.D. The Miracle of Fasting. Santa Barbara, CA: Bragg Health Sciences, 2004. E-book available at Bragg Health Products and Books. Accessed 29 May 2007 <www.bragg.com>.

EPA: United States Environmental Protection Agency. Accessed 2007-2008 <http://www.epa.gov>.

"Facts and Figures: Bottled Water." 2003 International Year of Fresh Water. 30 July 2003. UNESCO. <http://www.wateryear2003.org/en>.

GoGreenInStages.com. N.d. Accessed 2007-2008 <www.gogreeninstages.com>.

Kingston, Anne. "Green Report: It's So Not Cool." Macleans.ca. 14 May 2007. Maclean's Magazine. Accessed 2007-2008 <http://www.macleans.ca/article.jsp?content=20070514_105163_105163>.

Makino, Shinji, PhD. The Miracle of Pi-Water. Nagoya, Japan: IBE Company, 1994.

McRandle, P.W. "Plastic Water Bottles." The Green Guide. Mar/Apr. 2004. National Geographic. Accessed 2007-2008 <http://www.thegreenguide.com/doc/101/plastic>.

Mercola, Joseph, Dr., and Kendra Degen Pearsall. Sweet Deception: Why Splenda, NutraSweet, and the FDA May Be Hazardous to Your Health. Nashville, TN: Thomas Nelson, Inc., 2006.

NSF: The Public Health and Safety Company. 2004. NSF International. Accessed 2007-2008 <www.nsf.org>.

Ogasawara, Sherry, Kyra Watter, Kerry Sherk, Linda Sampson, and Linda Hutton. Nutrition and Wellness Specialist Certification Manual, 2nd ed. Markham, ON: Can-Fit-Pro, July 2002.

Parrot, Kathleen, Blake Ross, and Janice Woodard. Household Water Treatment. Publication. No. 356-481: May 1999. Virginia Cooperative Extension. Accessed 2007-2008 <http://www.ext.vt.edu/pubs/housing/356-481/356-481.html>.

PlasticFreeBottles.com. N.d. Accessed 2007-2008 <www.plasticfreebottles.com>.

PlasticInfo. N.d. Accessed 2007-2008 <www.plasticinfo.org>.

"Questions and Answers on Bottled Water." Health Canada. 7 Aug. 2007. Accessed 2007-2008 <http://www.hc-sc.gc.ca/fn-an/securit/facts-faits/faqs_bottle_water-eau_embouteillee-eng.php>.

Sizer, Frances, and Ellie Whitney. Nutrition Concepts and Controversies. 7th ed. Belmont, CA: Wadsworth Publishing Co., 1997.

Smith, Elizabeth, M.D. "Xenoestrogen: The Cause of Fibrocystic Breast Disease – How to Avoid Xenoestrogens." Fibrocystic Breast Disease. Accessed 4 Mar. 2007 <http:/www.fibrocystic.com/xeno.htm>.

Water Filter Comparisons. N.d. Doss Holdings Inc. Accessed 2007-2008 <www.waterfiltercomparisons.net>.

"Water Treatment Devices for Disinfection of Drinking Water." Health Canada. 28 Aug. 2008. Accessed 2008 <http://www.hc-sc.gc.ca/ewh-semt/pubs/water-eau/disinfect-desinfection-eng.php>.

Whang, Sang. AlkaLife. 2007. AlkaLife International. Accessed 29 May 2007 <www.alkalife.com>.

Whang, Sang. Reverse Aging. Miami, FL: JSP Publishing, 1990.

What's in Your Water? Pi-Mag Water Technology. Brochure. Irvine, CA: Nikken Inc., 2008.

WHO: World Health Organization. United Nations. Accessed 2007-2008 <http://www.who.int/en>.

Chapter 33: Boundaries – Stop! You Are In My Space

Cloud, Henry, and John Townsend. Boundaries, When to Say YES When to Say NO To Take Control of Your Life. Grand Rapids, MI: Zondervan, 1992.

Ford, Debbie. The Right Questions: Ten Essential Questions to Guide You to an Extraordinary Life. New York: Harper Collins, 2003.

Ford, Debbie. The Secret of the Shadow: The Power of Owning Your Whole Story. New York: Harper Collins, 2002.

Chapter 34: Cosmetics – Painting A Different Picture

"Cosmetics." U.S. Food and Drug Administration: Center for Food Safety and Applied Nutrition. U.S. Department of Health and Human Services. Accessed 2007-2008 <http://www.cfsan.fda.gov/~dms/cos-toc.html>.

"Cosmetic Products Ingredient Labelling." Health Canada. 19 Dec. 2006. Accessed 2007-2008 <http://www.hc-sc.gc.ca/iyh-vsv/prod/cosmet_prod_e.html>.

"Food, Nutrition, and Cosmetics: Questions and Answers." U.S. Food and Drug Administration: Center for Food Safety and Applied Nutrition. 29 Dec. 2006. U.S. Department of Health and Human Services. Accessed 2007-2008 <http://www.cfsan.fda.gov/~dms/qa-top.html>.

Hill, Aaron. "This Year Resolve to Update Cosmetics to Eco-Friendly Brand." Ewg.org (re-posted from Salem Monthly). 31 Dec. 2007. Environmental Working Group. Accessed 2007-2008 <http://www.ewg.org/node/25834>.

Johnson, Bonna. "Pucker Up: Industry Sees Rise in Organic Makeup." Ewg.org (re-posted from FloridaToday.com). 3 Jan. 2008. Environmental Working Group. Accessed 2007-2008 <http://www.ewg.org/node/25832>.

Mercola, Jospeph, Dr. "How Dangerous are Your Cosmetics?" Mercola.com. 17 July 2004. Dr. Joseph Mercola. Accessed 2007-2008 <http://articles. mercola.com/sites/articles/archive/2004/07/17/dangerous-cosmetics.aspx>.

Noll, Elizabeth. "Makeup Makeover: Natural Cosmetics Offer an Alternative to Toxic Beauty Products." Ewg.org (re-posted from Minnesota Women's Press). 25 Jan. 2006. Environmental Working Group. Accessed 2007-2008 <http://www.ewg.org/node/18357>.

Skin Deep: Cosmetic Safety Database. N.d. Environmental Working Group. Accessed 2007-2008 <www.ewg.org/reports/skindeep2>.

Soref, Anna. "Beautiful You: Natural Makeup Goes High End." Ewg.org (re-posted from Better Nutrition). 1 Feb. 2005. Environmental Working Group. Accessed 2007-2008 <http://www.ewg.org/node/16954>.

Swords, Tara. "Mineral Makeup: It's Trendy and Touted as All-Natural. But Does That Make it Good for You? Maybe." Ewg.org (re-posted from FloridaToday.com). 6 June 2006. Environmental Working Group. Accessed 2007-2008 <http://www.ewg.org/node/18690>.

The Campaign for Safe Cosmetics. Safe Cosmetics Action Network. Accessed 2007-2008 <www.safecosmetics.org>.

"The Ugly Face of our Cosmetics." Ewg.org (re-posted from Western Daily Press). 29 Aug. 2006. Environmental Working Group. Accessed 2007-2008 <http://www.ewg.org/node/18793>.

Chapter 38: Core Strength Simplified

McGill, Stuart. Ultimate Back Fitness and Performance. Waterloo, ON: Wabuno Publishers, 2004.

Chapter 41: Magnetism – What It Means To Us

Becker, Robert O., M.D., Cross Currents: The Promise of Electromedicine, the Perils of Electropollution. New York: Penguin Group, 1990.

Bloxham, Jeremy, and David Gubbins. "The Secular Variation of Earth's Magnetic Field." Nature (International Weekly Journal of Science). 317 (31 Oct. 1985): 777-781.

Bonlie, Dean. "How Magnetism Can Restore Energy and Health. Consumer Health Organization of Canada. 20.8 (Aug.1997). Accessed 16 Dec. 2007 <http://www.consumerhealth.org/articles/display.cfm?ID=19990303184500>.

Colbert, Agatha P., M.D., Marko S Markov, Ph.D., Mandira Baneiji, M.A. and Arthur A Pilla, Ph.D. "Magnetic Mattress Pad Use in Patients with Fibromyalgia: a Randomized Double-blind Pilot Study." Journal of Back and Musculoskeletal Rehabilitation. 13 (1999): 19-31.

Cox, Allen, "Magnetic Field Reversals", Scientific American, Feb. 1967, pp. 44-54.

Darendeliler, M., A. Darendeliler, and P. Sinclair. "Effects of Static Magnetic and Pulsed Electromagnetic Fields on Bone Healing." International Journal of Adult Orthodontic and Orthognathic Surgery. 12.1 (1997): 43-53.

Hall, Joe. "The Negative Effects of Electromagnetic Fields." 20.9 (Sep. 1997). Accessed 16 Dec. 2007 <http://www.consumerhealth.org/articles/display. cfm?ID=19990303201129>.

Hinman, M.R., J. Ford, and H. Heyl. "Effects of Static Magnets on Chronic Knee Pain and Physical Function: a Double-Blind Study." Alternative Therapies in Health and Medicine. 2002 Jul-Aug; 8.4 (Jul.-Aug. 2002): 50-5.

Huber, R., V. Treyer, A. A. Borbély, J. Schuderer, J. M. Gottselig, H.P. Landolt, E. Werth, T. Berthold, N. Kuster, A. Buck, and P. Achermann. "Electromagnetic Fields, such as those from Mobile Phones, Alter Regional Cerebral Blood Flow and Sleep and Waking EEG." Journal of Sleep Research. 11.4 (Dec. 2002): 289-95.

Gaudet, Pierre, M.Sc. Personal interviews. 2007-2008.

"Magnetic Research and Library Information." 5 Pillars – The eCommunity for Balanced Living. Accessed 3 Mar. 2008 <http://www.5pillars.com/ magneticresearch.cfm>.

Mercola, Joseph, Dr.. "Are EMFs Hazardous to Our Health?" Mercola.com. Dr. Joseph Mercola. Accessed 20 May 2008 <http://www.mercola.com/article/emf/ emf_dangers.htm>.

Ratterman R., J. Secrest, B. Norwood, and A.P. Ch'ien. "Magnet Therapy: What's the Attraction?" Journal of the American Academy of Nurse Practitioners. 14.8 (Aug. 2002): 347-353.

Thuile Ch., and M. Walzl. "Evaluation of Electromagnetic Fields in the Treatment of Pain in Patients with Lumbar Radiculopathy or the Whiplash Syndrome." NeuroRehabilitation. 17.1 (2002): 63-7.

Sher L. "The Effects of Natural and Man-Made Electromagnetic Fields on Mood and Behavior: The Role of Sleep Disturbances." Medical Hypotheses. 54.4 (Apr. 2000): 630-633.

Shimodaira, Kazuo, Dr. "Summary of a 12-month Double-Blind, Clinical Test of Magnetic Mattress Pads." Tokyo, Japan: Sanikukal Hospital, Tokyo Communications Hospital and Kouseikai Suzuki Hospital, 1990.

USA. Department of Health and Human Services. "Questions and Answers about Using Magnets to Treat Pain." National Centre for Complimentary and Alternative Medicine. May 2004. National Institutes of Health. Accessed 3 Mar. 2008 <http://nccam.nih.gov/health/magnet/magnet.htm#appendix2>.

Weintraub, Michael I., and Steven P. Cole. "Neuromagnetic Treatment of Pain in Refractory Carpal Tunnel Syndrome: An Electrophysiological and Placebo Analysis." Journal of Back and Musculoskeletal Rehabilitation. 15 (2000): 77-81.

Weintraub M.I., G.I. Wolfe, R.A. Barohn, S.P. Cole, G.J. Parry, G. Hayat, J.A. Cohen, J.C. Page, M.B. Bromberg, S.L. Schwartz, and the Magnetic Research Group. "Static Magnetic Field Therapy for Symptomatic Diabetic Neuropathy: a Randomized, Double-blind, Placebo-Controlled Trial." Archives of Physical Medicine and Rehabilitation. 84.5 (May 2003): 736-46.

Xu S., H. Okano, C. Ohkubo. "Acute Effects of Whole-body Exposure to Static Magnetic Fields and 50-Hz Electromagnetic Fields on Muscle Microcirculation in Anesthetized Mice." Bioelectrochemistry. 53.1 (Jan. 2001): 127-35.

Chapter 43: Beauty Sleep

"33 Secrets to a Good Night's Sleep." Mercola.com. N.d. Dr. Joseph Mercola. Accessed 5 May 2007 <http://www.mercola.com/article/sleep.htm>.

Ayas, Najib T., David P. White, JoAnn E. Manson, Meir J. Stampfer, Frank E. Speizer, Atul Malhotra, and Frank B. Hu. "A Prospective Study of Sleep Duration and Coronary Heart Disease in Women." Archives of Internal Medicine. 163.2 (27 Jan. 2003): 205-209.

"Inadequate Sleep Affects Hormones Levels." Mercola.com. 3 Sep. 2000. Dr. Joseph Mercola. Accessed 5 May 2007 <http://articles.mercola.com/sites/articles/archive/2000/09/03/sleep-hormones.aspx>.

Mercola, Joseph, Dr., with Rachael Droege. "Want to Prevent Cancer? Make Sure You Sleep Well." Mercola.com. 22 Oct. 2003. Dr. Joseph Mercola. Accessed 5 May 2007 <http://articles.mercola.com/sites/articles/archive/2003/10/22/cancer-sleep.aspx>.

Naska, Androniki, PhD; Eleni Oikonomou, BS; Antonia Trichopoulou, MD; Theodora Psaltopoulou, MD; and Dimitrios Trichopoulos, MD. "Siesta in

Healthy Adults and Coronary Mortality in the General Population." Archives of Internal Medicine. 167.3 (12 Feb. 2007): 296-301.

Schernhammer, Eva S., Bernard Rosner, Walter C. Willett, Francine Laden, Graham A. Colditz, and Susan E. Hankinson. "Epidemiology of Urinary Melatonin in Women and Its Relation to Other Hormones and Night Work." Cancer Epidemiology, Biomarkers & Prevention. Vol. 13 (June 2004): 936-943.

"Sleep Well to Live Well." Mercola.com. N.d. Dr. Joseph Mercola. Accessed 5 May 2007. <www.mercola.com>.

Sobel, David S., M.D. "One of the Best Cures for Insomnia." Mercola.com. 7 May 2000. Dr. Joseph Mercola. Accessed 5 May 2007 <http://articles.mercola. com/sites/articles/archive/2000/05/07/cure-insomnia.aspx>.

USA. Department of Health and Human Services. "Your Guide to Healthy Sleep." National Institutes of Health. Nov. 2005. National Heart, Lung, and Blood Institute. NIH Publication No. 06-5271. Accessed 2007-2008 <http:// www.nhlbi.nih.gov/health/public/sleep/healthy_sleep.pdf>.

USA. Department of Health and Human Services. "Brain Basics: Understanding Sleep." National Institute of Neurological Disorders and Stroke. 21 May 2007. National Institutes of Health. NIH Publication No. 06-3440-c. Accessed 2007-2008 <http://www.ninds.nih.gov/disorders/brain_basics/ understanding_sleep.htm#for_us>.

Vgontzas, A.N., E. Zoumakis, E.O. Bixler, H.M. Lin, H. Follett, A. Kales and G.P. Chrousos. "Adverse Effects of Modest Sleep Restriction on Sleepiness, Performance, and Inflammatory Cytokines." The Journal of Clinical Endocrinology & Metabolism. 89.5 (May 2004): 2119-2126.

Chapter 44: Cookware Awareness

"Enameled Cast Iron Cookware – Better Alternative for Healthy Cooking." Mercola.com N.d. Dr. Joseph Mercola. Accessed 15 May 2007. <www. mercola.com>.

LifeWare: Revolutionary Cookware. Accessed 2007-2008 <http://www.lifeware. us/index.html>.

"The Safe Use of Cookware." Health Canada. June 2006. Accessed 15 May 2007 <http://www.hc-sc.gc.ca/iyh-vsv/prod/cook-cuisinier_e.html>.

Woods, Rebecca. "Healthy Cookware." Be Nourished with Rebecca Wood. Accessed 2007-2008 <http://www.rwood.com/Articles/Healthy_Cookware. htm>.

Chapter 45: Guilt Is Eating You Up!

Ford, Debbie. The Right Questions: Ten Essential Questions to Guide You to an Extraordinary Life. New York: Harper Collins, 2003.

Chapter 46: What Is Wellness Chiropractic?

Creating Wellness™ Alliance. Conference notes & practitioner resources. Accessed 2006-2008 <www.creatingwellness.com>.

Feuling, Timothy J. Chiropractic works! Adjusting to a Higher Quality of Life. San Diego, CA: Wellness Solutions, 1999.